# The Natural Process of
# Quitting Forever:
## Explicit Instruction

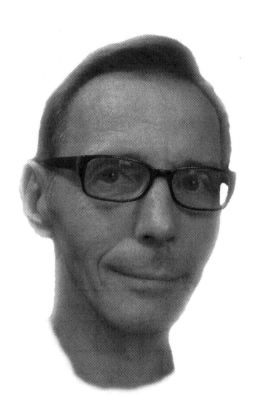

Take what we are talking about and don't use me as an authority. Think of what I am talking about and then question it. If it makes sense then you have made sense of it because it fits with reality. It is not my authority we are going by. If I say it is noon time so the sun is out, that has nothing to do with my authority, it is just that way. It is a fact. That is the way I am talking. Once you get the logic of it, you can figure it out yourself, because you have to do it yourself. Everyone who abstains does it themselves. You get the credit if you use drugs or drink alcohol. It is something you have done. The question is are you happy with what you have done by drinking or using? If you are happy with what you did then that helps explain why you are doing it again. Do you want to do it again? Well if you are happy with the results and want to do it again, that is why it is happening. It is only if you are not happy with what you have done, and you don't want to do it again. After that, we have something to talk about. I am not talking against what you want to have happen. You have your values. You decide how you want it to be. You decide what you want to have happen and then we can talk about how to accomplish it. It may seem like this is between me and you, but it is really between you, your values, and what you do.

*AuthorHouse™*
*1663 Liberty Drive, Suite 200*
*Bloomington, IN 47403*
*www.authorhouse.com*
*Phone: 1-800-839-8640*

*First published by AuthorHouse 1/14/2009*

*ISBN: 978-1-4343-9776-8 (sc)*

*Library of Congress Control Number: 2009900158*

*Printed in the United States of America*
*Bloomington, Indiana*

*This book is printed on acid-free paper.*

*www.quittingforever.org*
*MFT# 0602*
*LADC# 00464*

authorHOUSE®

# Table of Contents

# Introduction

If alcohol or drugs are causing you a problem, or even if you use but do not see a problem, and you decide it is time for quitting forever, then you want to end all alcohol and/or drug use. When people try to quit, many succeed without assistance and never use alcohol or drugs again as the result of a natural process they figure out through trial and error. You may find quitting forever was more difficult than you anticipated. If you go to self-help books, self-help groups, or a counselor or therapist, you likely will not find what you were looking for. The majority of self-help books are not about quitting forever. Counselors who write them have been trained in one-day-at-a-time, twelve-step approaches, relapse prevention, and some kind of therapy—cognitive, behavioral, interpersonal, or eclectic—to solve problems that they say may lead you to drink or use drugs.

What you are reading is explicit information on quitting the use of alcohol and drugs without returning to their use. If you want to make a permanent exit from alcohol/drug use, you can be quitting forever instead of going one day at a time. You do not have to wait until you feel like drinking or using to know what you are going to do. You do not have to run from the presence of alcohol or drugs, or worry about thinking about or feeling like using or drinking. You do not have to wait to solve personal problems or for spiritual divine intervention before quitting forever. You do not have to change all your friends before quitting forever. Quitting forever can be something you do first. Life changes you make are more easily discovered, because they support quitting forever. After quitting forever, the changes to be made follow naturally, because permanent abstinence promotes growth, eliminates self-defeating drinking and drugging and leads to the discovery of the other things that require changing.

If you have not thought about quitting forever and continue to drink or use drugs, that explains why you continue. If you have thought about quitting forever but have not done it, you have not yet truly made up your mind. You are ambivalent to quitting forever; you want to change, but you also want to get loaded again. You likely were not talked with about how to quit forever as a skill that works in all environments wherever you are and wherever you go. You may believe you have a disease that makes you drink or use when you do not want to. You may have been told—and believe—that quitting forever is not possible. You were on the right track if you thought about quitting forever and now want to carry it out. You can stop all alcohol and/or drug use and not return.

Quitting forever is real and attainable. Write down on paper your intention of quitting forever. It is time to make a plan. When will you have your last drink or drug? Can you stop without going into detox, or will you require assistance getting all the alcohol and drugs out of your system? Now, whom will you associate with now that you no longer drink alcohol or use drugs? What do you do when you think about or feel like using? Will you require medication to assist your body?

What do you do if you change your mind and drink or drug again? How do you stick with it until you make a permanent exit from further alcohol and drug use? How do you know that you have made a permanent exit from future alcohol and drug use? Only you can know when you are done with drinking and/or drugging. And, only you can carry out the natural process necessary to quit forever. No one can force you. No one can make quitting forever something you have to do. But, you can. And, it is your responsibility.

What I am talking about is different than much that has been written. There are similarities, because I have learned a lot from people who have criticized the twelve steps and recovery movement involved with them. Certainly, I am not the only one who talked about how to quit using alcohol and drugs forever. But, my criticism of the twelve steps and recovery movement is not just to validate those who have been wronged and deceived by those who dominate the alcohol and drug treatment arena. My intent is not to criticize the organizations on a total scale, but to pick out unhelpful statements and advice that run counter to quitting forever.

My criticism focuses distinctly on recovery advice that has become the folklore of help. I say folklore, because if you talk to the average person in America, when asked what to do if someone has an alcohol or drug problem, he or she will likely quote the twelve-step cliché, "One-day at a time and once an alcoholic/addict always an alcoholic/addict." The folklore permeate treatment in America, and few get help for an alcohol or drug issue without being referred to Alcoholics Anonymous (AA) or Narcotics Anonymous (NA). If no one has the courage to go over the destructive folklore point by point, the folklore lingers in the mind of the one trying to quit forever and plants the seeds of relapse and loss of control with catchy affirmations. Following the instructions of AA and NA leaves you living life in the identity of a second-class citizen, forever separated from others. You're afraid to go places they freely enter, because you are afraid drunkenness will overtake you. So, my criticism can help you deprogram from the information AA, NA, and disease-model counselors have planted in your mind. You can think for yourself and regain control over your hands and your life. Part of your brain may have been affected, but you can use a different part of your brain to abstain.

You see, the disease-concept counselors in the recovery movement have omitted important information that will aid you in ending your alcohol and drug problem. And, they assist in the deception by insisting religious activity is not religious activity when spiritual rituals are disguised as self-help activities.

The spiritual rituals are for the purpose of evoking a supernatural power to change your character. Spiritual rituals are not part of direct cause and effect in the natural world. Help from a supernatural power is not self-help but supernatural help. When you do the spiritual ritual in a twelve-step group or with your sponsor, you have to wait for the supernatural being to assist you. You do not directly take action; you do so indirectly, through something else. The directions you get are not direct and explicit, but are murky and confusing, and it is hard to understand what all this has to do with quitting alcohol or drugs.

Furthermore, universities and recovery centers withhold the information that there is a permanent exit from alcohol and drug abuse. They distort the model of recovery and leave out a permanent exit option from the recovery model so that it does not conflict with twelve-step folklore of endless relapses and an unpredictable drug and alcohol future. That is not all they leave out. When they teach you how alcohol and drugs affect a part of your brain, they conceal how voluntary movement comes from a different part of your brain. People spend thousands of dollars on treatment and understand why they desire to use again and again, but they never learn reasons how they can keep themselves from using. These omissions deserve criticism, since not teaching that information results in so much human suffering.

The best you get from the recovery movement is the development of motivational interviewing techniques that work on your own motivation to solve the problem and help you build on this motivation until you are alcohol and drug free. Motivational interviewing works as well as twelve-step recovery, but it is highly non-directive and does not provide information on quitting forever. Motivational interviewing helps a person work on making important choices and decisions, but does not teach someone how to make a choice or a decision. Motivational interviewing does not teach what a choice or decision is and does not show the difference between the two concepts. Motivational interviewing is when you ponder and wander with the help of a therapist until you figure out what to do. Substance abuse counselors and therapists teach a model of change but often leave out the concept of permanent exit as originally written by the authors of the model. The model of how to change taught by motivational interviewing is not a model of quitting forever.

I reemphasize: these omissions of information deserve criticism, as does the folklore of the twelve-step movement. The criticism is not for the purpose of deriding recovery programs, but for the purpose of telling people how to deprogram from harmful information they received and how to incorporate helpful information that has been withheld from them.

Get ready to learn what to do and what not to do, because I have written explicit instruction about how to move from choice to decision. If your decision is to quit forever the use of alcohol and drugs, here is explicit information about how to carry it out.

I have written about how to quit forever. I have not written about how to quit by solving personal problems, improving interpersonal relationships, or what you must do with your life before you are no longer drinking or drugging. Solving personal problems is something you do after quitting forever. You do not solve problems to quit forever, because that is bargaining about that act of permanently ending alcohol and drug use. Solving problems is an indirect method of recovery from alcohol and drug use, because it does not show you a natural method of quitting forever. Instead, problem solving assumes if you make your life better, then you will stop self-medicating with alcohol or drugs. The assumption ignores the fact that alcohol and drugs produce feelings of pleasure regardless of whether or not someone has problems. Alcohol and drugs are often used to make happy feelings more pleasurable. Some people drink alcohol and use drugs because they do not have problems; they just enjoy the effects of the substances.

Why wait? Quit now and get on with making your life better. Or, realize that you do not want to quit forever and drink/drug because that is your plan and intent to continue drinking and drugging, not because you are the helpless victim of a disease. Then, when some of the heath, emotional, financial, legal, and interpersonal problems associated with drinking and drug use befall you, you have no one to blame but yourself; then you might reconsider quitting forever. Either way, I believe it is better than being trapped in the recovery movement going to endless twelve-step groups.

# Quitting Forever
## Explicit Instructions

### 1. Think about quitting forever:

Do I really want to quit forever?

### 2. Intend on quitting forever:

When will I be quitting forever?

### 3. Decide on quitting forever:

Have I really done it?

### 4. Maintain Abstinence:

How many reasons do I need to abstain?

### 5. Permanent Exit:

How do I know I am done with it?

### 6. Deliberating:

Am I still debating reasons with myself while I wait to drink or use drugs?

# History of Quitting Forever

I talked to people about quitting forever before I was licensed as an alcohol and drug abuse counselor twelve years ago. I have always been talking and listening to people who continued permanent exit from further alcohol and drug use after quitting forever on their own.

I studied the Twelve Steps of Alcoholics Anonymous (AA) and could never buy into it. They seemed unbelievable to me. The groups seemed counterproductive. The one-day-at-a-time approach seemed like a promise to be able to drink or drug again, which was little more than one-delay-at-a-time. I learned relapse prevention and counseled people on using it. People who were not drinking or drugging told me that was not the way they were doing it. Rational Emotive Behavioral Therapy was showing ways to abstain without attending twelve-step groups and was among the first to point out that the twelve steps were religious activity.

Rational Recovery was an offshoot from Rational Emotive Behavioral Therapy. I became involved in Rational Recovery due to my training at the Institute on Rational Emotive Therapy (RET), now called the Albert Ellis Institute. For about seven years, I provided free Rational Recovery groups in the community, talking to people about their problems with being forced to attend twelve-step groups. People would stop using alcohol and drugs. I pointed out the fact anyone could keep themselves from drinking or using drugs. The question was how long they want to carry it out.

I received an opportunity to be paid to talk to people about Rational Recovery. I started offering groups in my private practice. One of the problems I kept having in both the free and paid sessions was that people came to me not knowing we were talking about lifelong abstinence. They heard incorrectly that Rational Recovery was about controlled drinking. They thought they would be joining a group of people to make friends. People did not always understand I was talking about quitting forever when they came to Rational Recovery.

I had other problems with Rational Recovery. Rational Recovery became as dogmatic as the recovery groups they were criticizing. Rational Recovery became exclusive with the corporate name and buzzwords like AVRT and the Beast. Rational Recovery ended all free recovery groups in the community and actively pursued anyone using the name Rational Recovery threatening legal action if they did not stop. They became critical of counselors and stopped trying to influence recovery in America. Rational Recovery morphed into an Internet website people pay to enter. Rational Recovery is not influenced by discoveries made from research and no longer teaches others how to talk to people about quitting the use of alcohol and drugs. Rational Recovery no longer attempts to defend those forced to attend twelve-step groups in violation of their First Amendment right of freedom of religion.

Quitting Forever has its roots in Rational Emotive Behavior Therapy and Rational Recovery, but I was enlightened by talking to people about the process of quitting forever, while being influenced by current research validating quitting forever without the use of twelve-step groups and moving beyond relapse prevention. The sacred cows that oppose the ability of people to make a permanent exit from alcohol and drug abuse are questioned using rational and critical thinking. Logical contradictions of the recovery movement are the focus of Quitting Forever questions and answers. Written with an attempt to use the language without made-up buzzwords from the recovery movement, Quitting Forever reviews reasons why anyone can abstain from alcohol and drugs for the remainder of one's life.

It is now known a decision is the starting point. The skills one uses to decide before quitting forever are different than the skills it takes after quitting forever. How do you move from choice to decision? What do you do after you decide to quit forever?

Research and what to do were there but not put together until Quitting Forever. You have the opportunity to determine where you are in the process of quitting forever. You get to review your motivation to drink and drug and review your motivation to abstain from alcohol and drugs. You have the opportunity to witness yourself going back and forth between wanting it and wanting to avoid it. You can start to see how alcohol and drugs became more important to you as your values changed. Your willingness to think about quitting forever is part of your intent.

There is a difference between forever choosing and making a decision based on your values. You will learn the difference between choosing and making a decision. Quitting Forever developed the model for teaching the difference between choosing and deciding. Knowing how to decide can help you make up your mind about what you want to do.

Quitting Forever is based on a biological model of using alcohol and drugs. The biological model is also the base for the disease concept of alcohol or drug use. But, the disease concept leaves many rational questions unanswered when it explains why you will always be sick. Quitting Forever show a "brain recovery model" that can be verified in any textbook on neuroanatomy. The brain recovery model explains why you can keep yourself from drinking or using drugs. It shows what happened to you is a natural result of consuming alcohol and/or drugs.

Quitting Forever brings forward advances in behavioral therapy you can apply to yourself after quitting forever. Once quitting forever is completed, it is time to stop choosing. There is no reason to avoid the thoughts and feelings to use or to fight them like a beast out to get you. Thoughts and feelings to use are the natural result of drinking and drugging. There is an alternative to avoiding or fighting them. You can gain a new confidence in your ability to abstain in the face of response tendencies to drinking alcohol and using drugs. You can stop being a second-class citizen and start living your life based on your values, solving problems for the solution not to keep yourself from drinking or drugging. You determine how much support you need to abstain and who will give you support. Most people get support from family, friends, church groups, and organizations. Associate with people because you like them not because they used to have an alcohol or drug problem. You will know what to do after quitting forever. What happened to you is a natural result of consuming alcohol and/or drugs.

# Consider The Dominant Advise

The Addiction and Recovery Organization in Canada provides advice on their website about relapse prevention. The organization provides techniques for dealing with mental urges to drink alcohol or use drugs. Doing your recovery one day at a time and distracting yourself are two of the relapse-prevention techniques they provide. It is the advice you will likely get if you seek counseling or go for treatment. The following is an examination of those techniques. Benefits and drawbacks of the techniques are examined.

## One Day at a Time

The explanation about using one day at a time is one of the best I have read. It is concise, and advice is easy to understand. It is both motivating and convincing. It is identical to advice twelve-step groups, substance abuse counselors, and rehabilitation centers tell clients. The following reference is a direct quote from the www.addictionandrecovry.org site:

*Don't think about whether you can stay abstinent forever. That's a paralyzing thought. It's overwhelming even for people who've been in recovery for a long time. One day at a time means you should match your goals to your emotional strength. When you feel strong and you're motivated to not use, then tell yourself that you won't use for the next week or the next month. But when you're struggling and having lots of urges, and those times will happen often, tell yourself that you won't use for today or for the next 30 minutes. Do your recovery in bite-sized chunks and don't sabotage yourself by thinking too far ahead.*

## Paralyzed: Possible Response to Abstinent Forever

Reread the first two sentences. They tell you that if you even think about quitting forever, you will become paralyzed and overwhelmed. Test what they have said by thinking about never drinking alcohol or using drugs again, and reflecting on your experience. You will see you are not paralyzed or overwhelmed. You will have a response to the thought of never drinking or using drugs again. What happens is you accept the idea or you refuse the idea. Next, I next review the different possible responses to the thought of quitting forever by never drinking or using drugs again.

You endorse the idea as relevant to solving your problem. When some people say in their heads like whispering words to themselves in the form of thinking, "*I will never use alcohol or drugs, ever,*" they say it sounds like a good idea. Some of those who see quitting forever as a good idea are motivated by the quick and powerful solution. The thought fills them with determination and hope.

1. At that point, some people decide, "It is a good idea for me. I quit forever. Now is as good a time as any to start. There will never be a better time than right now." And, they quit forever. They are determined to never use alcohol or drugs again and set on a course to carry out their decision.

2. Some people endorse the idea of quitting forever but think they do not want to quit right now. For some people, the idea of quitting forever becomes a reason why they should continue to drink alcohol or use drugs. They think, *"It is too long to go without drinking or drugging if I never do it again. I will do it some more before I quit."* Procrastination is when you put off something that could be done now. But, procrastination is not a paralyzed or overwhelmed response. If you were paralyzed or overwhelmed, you would not be able to plan anything. On the contrary, procrastination helps you plan your next drink or drug use.

3. Some people refuse the idea of never drinking or drugging ever. (a) They refuse the idea because they want to drink or drug again. (b) They refuse because they do not think that the act of quitting forever can be carried out. (c) And, they refuse because they do not think quitting forever is the best way to end alcohol or drug use.

3a. Some people do not like the idea of quitting forever, because they actively want to use alcohol or drugs again. Is that because they are addicted? Maybe, but if they detox, they are not under the influence of alcohol or drugs. But, the aftereffects of using of alcohol or drugs affected their brain. They know how good it feels to use alcohol or a drug and want to return to the feeling by drinking or using again. This is the point where the trouble with addiction enters. How is it known the person is addicted and not that they just want to drink or use again as a matter of preference? Addictionologists point to brain studies that show changes in brain chemistry they say account for why the person wants to drink or drug again. But, what they cannot account for is why some people with identical drinking or drugging profiles decide on quitting forever after thinking about never drinking or using drugs again.

3b. Some people refuse the idea of quitting forever, because they do not think it can be carried out. Any human being just can't —at least not someone who is an alcoholic or addict. Those unfortunate people lack education. They do not understand the neurology of how voluntary movement takes place. They could be educated to understand that feeling like using alcohol or drugs is the result of past use and is not the sole cause of future use. Neurology shows the part of the brain affected with the aftereffects of alcohol or drug use and desire is not the part of the brain that controls the arms and hands. Feeling like using does not mean one is an alcoholic. Using the terms alcoholic and addict as self-identifiers or labels is not helpful when explaining why you do something. It is not logical thinking.

3c. The one-day-at-a-time motto is dominant in the drug and alcohol recovery industry. The drug and alcohol recovery network largely ignores people quitting forever, because people quitting forever have done it outside formal alcohol and drug treatment programs. The alcohol and drug recovery network continues to present one day at a time as the only way to recovery when it is but one option. The quitting forever option is never mentioned in treatment. When a person in treatment independently brings up the idea of quitting forever, counselors carry out their training and say, "Don't think about whether you can stay abstinent forever." If a person mentions quitting forever to their twelve-step group, members chant, "One day at a time," and openly criticize. Everyone in the group hears the criticism repeated, and they are influenced to believe one day at a time is the only way to keep from drinking or using drugs.

## Return to critical analysis of the remaining sentences:

*One day at a time means you should match your goals to your emotional strength. When you feel strong and you're motivated to not use, then tell yourself that you won't use for the next week or the next month. But when you're struggling and having lots of urges, and those times will happen often, tell yourself that you won't use for today or for the next 30 minutes. Do your recovery in bite-sized chunks and don't sabotage yourself by thinking too far ahead.*

## Match Your Goals to Your Emotional Strength

I agree with the statement that one should match goals to their emotional strength. Imagine what one day at a time does to someone's emotional strength compared to when they think quitting forever is a good idea. The person being told one day at a time is being told they do not have the emotional strength to quit forever. There is no assessment to determine if the person has the emotional strength. Lack of emotional strength is assumed due to the recovery industry's endorsement of one day at a time. A mismatch has taken place between the person quitting forever and the advice-giver: the goal is not matched to the emotional strength as advised. The advice-giver discourages the intention to end alcohol and drug use forever with an idea that it cannot be done. Instead, people who think about quitting forever can be shown how it can be done and, if carried out, guarantees intoxication from alcohol or drugs will never happen again. If you are thinking about quitting forever, the presence of the thought is indication you have the emotional strength.

Think about the uncertainty of not using alcohol or drugs only for a while. When you are struggling and having lots of urges, you think about not using in bite-sized chunks of thirty minutes to a month. The advice seems like a good idea. But, it entails the idea alcohol and drug use should not be ended. Someone thinking about not using for thirty days is comforted by the idea they can use in thirty days. Not using for thirty minutes entails being able to use in thirty minutes. At the end of thirty minutes, you again think of not using for another thirty minutes or, if you are stronger, not using for thirty days. And, not drinking does not have to bother you, because you can always drink in thirty days. And, in thirty days, you can always choose to not drink for another thirty minutes or thirty days. You play an endless trick on yourself. No wonder relapse rates are so high. You know it is just a trick you are playing, and now that you made day thirty, you can go and drink or use drugs again.

One day at a time weakens emotional strength when emotional strength should be sustained with support. You think about quitting forever, and you are told one day at a time. If you believe them, you believe you do not have the strength for quitting forever, though you actually do have it. You will not use the emotional strength you have, and it will be as though you are emotionally weak. When you feel like drinking or using, one-day-at-a-time will create a struggle, because you will be telling yourself, "I will not drink now. I will wait until later." Waiting to drink or use drugs creates a struggle. Judging by relapse statistics, it is a struggle most people frequently lose. It is frustrating to have to wait.

Quitting forever builds emotional strength, because it stops choosing and ends the struggle. When you feel like drinking or using drugs, you know quitting forever has taken place. There is nothing to consider after quitting forever. You feel like drinking or drugging, but you know that is done. You don't have to wait thirty minutes or thirty days to drink or drug again because of quitting forever. You know the feeling to drink or drug was caused by past drinking or drugging in the past, and it is not your intent to drink or use drugs again. Your hands and arms won't move to pick up alcohol or drugs unless you make them do that. You quit forever. There is no reason to pick up alcohol or drugs. The feeling will go away if you don't drink for a while or if you never drink again. You are not waiting, and you feel less frustrated than one day at a time.

Research explains what happens to someone who expects to do something again when they have the feeling to do it, compared to those who accept they will never do it again. The feeling lasts longer in those who expect to do something again compared to those who expect they will never do it again. Expecting something to happen again means you are not doing it while you wait to do it. Waiting to do something is the definition of frustration. It is more frustrating to wait for something you might do again than to give up waiting. Waiting is frustrating. Accepting you will no longer do something is much less frustrating. Accepting you quit ends waiting. And, it become less frustrating the more you accept it. Accepting does not have to take a long time. Some people take to it quite naturally. It is easier to accept you will no longer drink or use drugs by quitting forever than it is to go one-day-at-a-time, saying you won't do it for now but maybe later.

> # Alcohol and drug use is one day at a time.
> # If you do not use again, you sober up and are clean.

## How Will You Be Paralyzed?

I question how the thought of never drinking or using drugs again would paralyze someone. *Merriam Webster*'s dictionary defines paralyze as, "inability to move or a state of powerlessness." I doubt the Addiction and Recovery Organization meant someone would be literally paralyzed. Were they using paralyzed as a figure of speech, meaning you would be unable to move forward in your recovery? Recovery is about never using again. How could thinking about a solution leave someone unable to move forward to the solution of never drinking again?

In reality, avoiding the thought of quitting forever is paralyzing. You sabotage your recovery with one-day-at-a-time. It makes you unable to move forward in your recovery. One-day-at-a-time sets up endless waiting to drink or use again, while you tell yourself, "Not now. I will wait thirty minutes before I drink or use." Instead, you could be using your emotional strength of confidence knowing about your quitting forever. You are not waiting to drink or drug. You make room for the feeling to drink or use. You are not afraid of the feeling, because you expected it would happen because of the fact that you drank or used a drug. You know you decided on quitting forever, and there is no drink or drug to wait for. Knowing you are not ever going to use, you can go on and focus on activities before you and follow your values.

## Distraction is Secondary

The Addiction and Recovery Organization advises you to use distraction, but they rob you of the opportunity to think about quitting forever with one-day-at-a-time. When something is resolved in your mind, you have a way to think about it. One-day-at-a-time keeps you from resolving the issue of whether you are going to drink alcohol or use drugs. If you just distract yourself, you are not facing the responsibility to yourself to decide whether you will ever drink or use drugs again. The feeling to use will go away with just using distraction, but with one-day-at-a-time, you will never be sure if you will again intoxicate yourself with alcohol or drugs. One-day-at-a-time distraction is first because you distract yourself from drinking or using by just getting through the day.

Quitting forever makes distraction come second. You know you are never going to drink or use drugs again, but you also know you feel like drinking or using. You are confident you are not going to drink or drug because of quitting forever. You accept any feelings or thoughts you have about drinking. Thoughts and feelings to drink are not a sign of relapse after quitting forever. They signal what your drinking and drugging have done to you. They will become less bothersome because of never drinking or drugging again. You accept them as they are right now. Procrastinating your drinking or drug use will only make the feeling last longer and be stronger. Quitting forever will get you through.

Quitting forever will let the feelings to use go, because you never drink or use drugs. It is just a matter of time. You look forward to the next thirty minutes or next thirty days, because you know you will not drink or use drugs. You do not trick yourself by looking forward to a time when you can drink or use again to get through the right now. Procrastinating your drinking or drug use will only make the feeling last longer and be stronger. Quitting forever will get you through. You can depend on yourself. You are the best person to run your life. Start doing what you want, knowing you will not be drinking or using drugs.

---

> # There is a difference between no thoughts to drink or drug and a decision to never drink and drug.

---

## Is Quitting Forever too Easy or too Hard?

I have criticized one day at a time. I conclude with addressing criticism about quitting forever. Quitting forever does not mean someone will not be able to change his or her mind and drink or drug again. Quitting forever sets up internal conditions to make the use of alcohol or drugs more difficult. It is more difficult, because you have to tell yourself to drink after you told yourself you would never drink. And, you set your course on quitting forever because of your values. It was important to you. Even if someone drinks or drugs again, it is easier for them to determine how they changed their mind if they continue their conviction of quitting forever. As with cigarettes, those who keep quitting until they get it right change their behavior. When carried out, quitting forever provides permanent exit from the alcohol/drug use relapse cycle.

Quitting forever is too easy. Quitting forever is just easy to understand. It can be difficult to make up your mind about quitting forever, but once your mind is made up, not drinking or using drugs is not difficult. It is easier to go one-day-at-a-time than to make the decision about quitting forever. However, quitting forever carried to its natural conclusion is much more effective and much easier than going one-day-at-a-time.

# Informed Consent:
# Reasons Why You May Not Want to Read *Quitting Forever*

*Quitting Forever* is about just what the name means: quitting alcohol and drugs for the remainder of your life. It means abstaining from both alcohol and drugs for as long as you live. It provides explicit information about quitting forever and how to carry it out. *Quitting Forever* attacks ideas that go against the idea of quitting forever. It attacks ideas that convince you not to quit forever, because believing those ideas can keep you addicted. Why would anyone want to keep you addicted is beyond me, and I will not speculate why.

There is much misinformation and deception in the recovery movement. *Quitting Forever* is about getting out of the recovery movement, because you don't need it anymore. Why would you need the recovery movement—or any part of it—if you never use alcohol or drugs again? You would look, sound, and act no different than anyone else who did not use, and there are plenty of us. There are the people who never used. There are people who used some and don't anymore; there are people who used a lot, and fell in love with it, who don't use anymore. There is no way to tell these people apart if they don't reveal their drinking or drug history. You would be no different then any of them. They all have their own unique set of problems that make them human. Problems don't make people drink or use drugs.

When I write that problems don't make people drink or use drugs, that statement is one of the reasons you may not want to read *Quitting Forever*. *Quitting Forever* will tell you things that are contrary to the recovery movement. Reading *Quitting Forever* may put you at odds with your current therapist, counselor, or drug rehab person. They are likely all representatives of the twelve-step AA and NA groups and the recovery movement in general. They are well-meaning people and are well trained to teach you that you have a disease, that you cannot quit forever, and that you have problems you need help with to keep from drinking or using drugs. Be forewarned: reading *Quitting Forever* can hurt your relationship with therapists, college professors, medical doctors, and psychiatrists. There is a psychiatrist in Reno, Nevada, who openly advocates withholding needed medication from people who refuse to attend twelve-step groups. Your doctor may withhold medical treatment you need for your health to get you to go.

One of the problems with reading *Quitting Forever* is that you may hold yourself responsible for you past, present, and future drugging and/or drinking. You may regret what you have done and have no one to blame for it anymore. You may not have reasons to relapse and may not even believe in the concept of slips and relapses when it comes to the use of alcohol and drugs. Quitting forever may not be something you want to do. It has some drawbacks in that you will never get drunk or high again if you carry it out. The recovery movement and the twelve steps hold a better offer for those who don't want to face life without sometimes getting loaded.

The recovery movement doesn't teach about quitting forever. They teach you one day at a time and one urge at a time with relapse prevention. Both of these are a great bargain for future drinking and drugging. With a disease, it will not be your fault when you relapse and slip back into addiction. You can say you stopped treatment or did not work a good step. You learned some great excuses that you will no longer use after quitting forever.

The next time you drink or drug you can always use the slogan, "Relapse is part of recovery." Your counselor will understand what you are talking about and be happy to give you another assignment and really empathize with your illness. Go to your twelve-step group and sit in the back, like you are ashamed after you drank or drugged. Tell them you weren't working a good program. They will understand just what you mean and love you for it. You will have some great stories to share about your recent use. Tell the judge you drank or used but that you realized you really didn't do a good step 2 or 3 and that you got a different sponsor. The judge will say, "Good for you." Fake it until you make it. But, if you go and tell your counselor, recovery group, or the judge about Quitting Forever and wanting to end recovery help to get on with your life, they will be mad at you. You may be forced into ninety meetings in ninety days with strict monitoring

> # There is no easy way out.
> # Once you stop drinking and/or drugging,
> # the next question is for how long.

Better to go out and drink or use than tell the judge, your counselor, or your twelve step group about quitting forever. You may receive scorn, stern lectures, and outright scolding. You may be told that you are in the process of relapse by even suggesting someone could quit forever. Reading *Quitting Forever* will tell you how to quit forever and will critique those recovery ideas just presented. It will not only critique them, but it will provide you a way to counter your recovery-helping tormentors that may leave them angry and frustrated. The majority of counselors and therapists are in deep denial about people quitting forever, and as you break through some of their denial, they will feel anxiety and anger and may blame you for it.

You may not want to read further and hear the disease concept burst like a wet paper bag filled with water. It holds, but don't poke into it, or it may start to leak and then burst. The disease concept will be examined, because it keeps more people addicted than ever was intended. You may not want to find out the flaws in logic of the brain-disease concept or find out about the neurobiology of voluntary movement the recovery movement leaves out. Instead of the brain-disease model, you will learn the brain-recovery model by reading *Quitting Forever*. Finding out how you voluntarily continue to use alcohol and drugs may make you feel anxiety that you didn't stop sooner, and you may become angry at people who told you that you could never quit forever. You may think you have been lied to when you learn that the Twelve Steps of AA and NA are religious activities as defined by the Constitution of the United States, and that your alcohol and drug counselor was likely taught how to deceive you by receiving training from a college or university system with the deception known by their licensing board of examiners who may also be in twelve step groups. The Nevada Board of Nursing still forces nurses into twelve steps as a condition for keeping their license.

Furthermore, if you tell yourself you quit forever and go back on your word to yourself, it can have negative emotional ramifications. You may feel guilty that you drank or drugged again. You may feel ashamed of yourself. You may feel like you did wrong. You may feel anxiety about your drinking and drug use, and it may not be as much fun as before. You may feel like you are lying when you try to use your old excuses. You may never be able to return to an AA or NA meeting again. You may never want to talk to another alcohol or drug counselor again. And, your legal and financial problems may return.

After quitting forever, some of your family and friends may not approve. Relationships have broken up because one spouse quit forever while the other kept using. The using spouse wanted out of the relationship now that the partner was no longer relapsing. People who only had being high in common with you may no longer want to be around you when you refuse to drink or drug with them. And, none of them may ever believe you that you have quit forever. You may be the only one who knows about your quitting forever when you abstain.

Do not read any more unless you are ready to quit your alcohol and drug use forever. You can't get over your problems in alcohol- and drug-recovery groups. Get marriage and family or couples therapy to solve relationship problems. Go to groups to get psychological therapy to solve emotional or thinking problems. Get over it by getting on with life. You don't do anything to remain clean and sober. You remain clean and sober to do anything. Don't solve problems to stay clean and sober. Stay clean and sober to solve problems.

> *God grant me the serenity*
> *to accept the things I cannot change;*
> *courage to change the things I can;*
> *and wisdom to know the difference. Amen.*
>
> Reinhold Niebuhr

The Serenity Prayer was written for solders during World War II who did not know if they were going to live through the day. It was not written to encourage people to call themselves alcoholic or addict. It was not written to make someone believe they could not quit alcohol or drugs.

# Myth in Recovery

The Serenity Prayer of Reinhold Niebuhr is associated with AA and NA. But, it does not seem that God has blessed that organization or the recovery movement counselors with wisdom.

"Accept the things I cannot change." They want you to accept that you cannot change being addict or an alcoholic. "Courage to change the things I can" means you can stop drinking or using drugs just for today, for tomorrow, or forever. And, and the "wisdom to know the difference." The twelve-step and recovery movements, which include many substance abuse counselors, do not have the wisdom to know the difference. They were not taught the difference in their university courses, nor were they required to know the difference to become licensed. They are taught to perpetuate myth.

**Myth:** If you become addicted to a substance, then you are an alcoholic or an addict. When we are talking about rehabilitation, there is a concept known as role recovery. Role recovery is where you think of yourself as living an accepted role in your community no different and equal to other people living in your community. Living the role of alcoholic or addict is not role recovery but loss of normal identity. You give up your identity of everything else, and first become an alcoholic and addict. You keep that role forever. We know that many people who take on the label become worse and do worse. You do not have to call yourself anything to stop using alcohol or drugs. Think of yourself as a carpenter, writer, mother, father, sister, or brother. Think of yourself as anything but an alcoholic or an addict, and you will do better when it comes to ending your alcohol or drug problem.

**Myth**: Quitting one-day-at-a-time takes courage. Only stopping one-day-at-a-time is so you don't have to use the courage to face never using alcohol or drugs again, and you don't have to feel let down when you get drunk or loaded again because you never said you would not do it again. There is nothing to be afraid of in stopping just for today. You can always get loaded tomorrow. But, if there is nothing to be afraid of, then no courage is required, because it only takes courage to do something that is fearful. Besides, the recovery movement has taken the second part of the prayer, "Living one day at a time," and morphed it into only quitting one day at a time. They advocate one day at a time because they say you can never predict if you are going to drink or drug again in the future.

**Myth:** Twelve-step groups and recovery counselors do not have the wisdom to know the difference between what can and what cannot be done. The wisdom is that anyone who desires to quit forever the use of alcohol or drugs can do it if they know how to make the decision and carry it out. Those extolling one day at a time were not granted the wisdom to know that an alcohol or drug problem can be ended forever. They cannot teach you what they do not know. They do not have the wisdom to tell people about quitting forever. They believe it is something that cannot be done, when it can be done.

# Principles of Quitting Forever

1. **You can quit anytime you want.** If you are still drinking alcohol and/or using drugs, then you may or may not have thought about quitting. The thought about quitting forever may have never crossed your mind. If you thought about quitting, it may not have been carried beyond being a thought. You may have stopped, but you started again. Quitting forever is something that can be carried out anytime you're ready. Your ability to carry out quitting forever is a biological fact.

2. **You have both thoughts to drink and use drugs and thoughts to quit.** Think about your next drink or drug use. Do you want to continue as you have been doing? What comes to mind along with the good thoughts about drinking or using drugs? You know something should be done about what you have been doing. But, when you think about quitting forever, you start to think about drinking or using again. You can observe your mind going back and forth between drinking alcohol and using drugs and giving them up.

3. **Your mind is not made up, but it can be.** You may not have taken the time to think it through seriously. You may be confused about having both the thoughts to drink and use and to knock it off, because you do not have a way to understand what is going on. You do not have to stop one set of thoughts to make up your mind. You have values to tell you what to do. You are the one who determines what is right for you. You know what is the right thing for you to do.

4. **You can make a decision and stop choosing.** You don't know what your are going to do in the future when it comes to using drugs or drinking alcohol again. You will be forced to make a choice. You will do it again, or you will not do it again. You may be choosing again and again. Re-choosing is the problem. Your values are what you do. You can make a decision to follow your values no matter what you think or feel. You do not have to keep buying into thoughts to use.

5. **You can stop using reasons.** Reasons may be the place to start, but they are not the place to finish. Reasons keep you choosing. Reasons not to drink or drug usually entail reasons to drink or use drugs. You can talk your way out of doing it again for only so long. If you are using reasons, then your mind is not made up. Reasoning your way out of drinking or using means you have not made a decision to follow your values. You do not have to keep buying into thoughts to use.

6. **You are the best person to run your life.** You are not completely in control of what happens or the opportunities that will present themselves. You are in control of whether or not you will ever drink alcohol or use drugs again. If you are in a family, a relationship, or on the job, you may have people telling you what to do, but it is your choice to do what they want or what you want. If you do something and it does not turn out the way you want, then you have a better chance of doing it differently if you are not drinking or using drugs. Drinking and using drugs can become so important that getting loaded again is running your life. Then, you give people more chance to take advantage of you.

## Values Expressed in Quitting Forever

**Orientation on the Person.** When quitting forever, you are a person with existing strengths and abilities that will let you abstain from alcohol and drugs as long as you desire. The twelve steps label you as an alcoholic with no power. The recovery movement places you as a patient or a client.

**First Class Citizen.** When quitting forever, you focus on the real world. You face the fact that alcohol and drugs will be there for the asking, but you will never pick them up or use them. The twelve steps want you to hide from alcohol and drugs and mostly go to their groups. The recovery movement warns against being in slippery places like stores and restaurants where alcohol is served.

**Functioning.** When quitting forever, you abstain from alcohol and drugs, so of course you are sober. You focus on everyday activities and make changes in your life as you see necessary for your comfort and benefit. You do not make lifestyle changes to abstain. You abstain to make life changes. Both the twelve steps and the recovery movements warn against making any changes during the first year of sobriety. Sobriety means not drunk or high on drugs.

**Support.** When quitting forever, you realize that you do not need support to do the right or correct thing. What is supportive to one person is not supportive to the next. Associate with the people you can get along with because of common interests. You do not drink or use drugs anymore, and who you find supportive will come out of that. The twelve steps say you need both the support of AA and NA members, and you must have the support of a sponsor. The recovery movement thinks in terms of a support group.

**Involvement.** When you quit forever, it is your own involvement in abstaining that brings the result. Your active participation in using your ability to observe your drinking or using thoughts and feelings, and your ability to abstain in the face of them, is something you are confident doing. Your ability to abstain will work in all environments. The twelve steps tell you to keep coming back because it works. The recovery movement provides treatment that is supposed to work.

**Self Determination.** When quitting forever, you use self-determination and face your readiness to make a decision about your future use of alcohol and drugs forever. You are guided by your values, not your thoughts to use alcohol or drugs. The Twelve Steps *Big Book* repeatedly criticizes self-determination and labels it as being self-centered. The recovery movement may go to great lengths to counsel you to follow their treatment plans and follow the gradual path to recovery as a complex and time-consuming process.

**Outcome.** When quitting forever, you stop counting time since your last drink or drug use and abstain because of quitting forever. The process is you never drink or use drugs again, giving you the outcome of new direction based on your values. The twelve steps has a one-day-at-a-time outcome. You never know what you will do tomorrow, and therefore, you live a life of uncertainty. They have you celebrate sobriety birthdays and get chips. The recovery movement counts sobriety day by day. They also count the number of twelve-step meetings you attend by having you get your slip signed.

## Do You Want to Quit Using Alcohol and Drugs Forever?

I am interested in people who want to quit the use of alcohol and drugs forever and never use them again—no matter what happens or how they feel. I never thought there were people like that until I was involved in the underground recovery movement. Part of my discovery was described in the history of Quitting Forever. I have talked with people about quitting forever for over sixteen years. Most, but not all, refused to endorse the disease model or the twelve steps, but they were influenced. I discovered the influence was negative and actually prevented people from being fully confident they had reached their goal of quitting forever. They were left filled with doubt because of their treatment experience. The curious thing I began to notice was the more substance-abuse treatment and the more twelve-step meetings attended meant the person had more reasons why they should not quit forever. Discussions with people who wanted to quit forever but who were talked out of it by well-meaning counselors and twelve-step believers greatly influenced what I teach people today.

Does everyone want to quit forever? No, they do not. I am not trying to reach people who do not want to stop using forever. Do I want people to stop attending twelve-step groups and going one day at a time? No, I will refer anyone who wants to attend a twelve-step group and who cannot find one. I am interested in people who refuse twelve steps on their own. Am I telling people that they don't have a disease? Yes. You do not have a disease that makes you put alcohol or drugs in your body unless you want to put them there. Does putting alcohol or drugs in your body cause disease? Yes! Biological injuries created by alcohol and drugs in the human body are facts. But, the injuries created by alcohol and drugs do not make you use them again.

What happens is you want to use alcohol and drugs again, even though it caused injury, because alcohol and drugs make you feel pleasure and change your values. That is another biological fact. Alcohol and drugs stimulate a pleasure center in your brain. You use alcohol and drugs to stimulate that pleasure center. When you use alcohol and drugs again and again to a certain level of intoxication, you develop a hunger and a love for that feeling, and you want to return to it again and again. Alcohol and drugs become more important to you. You develop a response set to pick them up and use them again to get the reward of pleasure. Sure, you feel pain, but too long after the use for it to be a behavioral deterrent. You usually start to feel pain when not using.

Some people want to quit forever. They want to bring an end to their repeated self-intoxication. They do not want to solve life problems or engage in new religious rituals at first. They do not want to contact supernatural higher powers or work steps. They do not want to have a disease in which they relapse out of their own control. They do not want to live the remainder of their lives calling themselves alcoholics or addicts and going to groups. Plenty of people do not like the insecure feeling of one-day-at-a-time sobriety. They just want to quit using alcohol or drugs and not do it anymore. They don't need an assessment or anyone else to tell them they should quit forever. They just need a way to figure out how to do it themselves. Am I talking to you?

Do you know the moral/ethical principles involved in quitting forever? The old moral model was that you got drunk or used drugs to excess because you lacked moral fortitude. The old moral model was very blaming. The modern moral model is rational.

Is it right to use alcohol and drugs when you know they lower your value judgments? Alcohol and drugs change your values while you are loaded and after you sober up and are detoxed.

The moral stance toward alcohol and drug use was for the most part discontinued from use by counselors, therapists, AA/NA, and the recovery movement in general. The unfortunate side effect of dropping the moral model and starting a disease model left no place for moral reasoning when thinking about further use. There were no moral issues involved in getting a disease that makes you drink and use against your will. You complete a moral inventory in twelve steps, but the use of alcohol or drugs is not part of that inventory. They do not have you question and ponder if it is morally right for you to continue using alcohol or drugs.

You do not need to complete a fearless moral inventory, because we are only talking about one moral issue: whether or not it is right for you to drink alcohol and use drugs again after you know they change your values. There is a moral issue to be considered before taking your next drink or before you use your next drug. Is it right for you to do it again? We are not talking about what other people or the country should do.

Alcohol and drugs change your values. They change your values when you are under the influence and when you sober up. When you are under the influence of alcohol or drugs, you are disinhibited from doing things you would not do when sober. Your moral code is lowered under the influence. When you sober up and come off the alcohol or drugs, your values are changed. Using alcohol and drugs becomes more important to you than before. And, drugs and alcohol can become more important the more you return to getting high. They compete with your family and friends for your attention. They make it difficult to figure out the right thing to do. Drinking alcohol or using drugs becomes more important than doing other things. Or, doing other things without using alcohol or drugs becomes less important.

Using alcohol to excess does not mean you lack morals, although when you are high on alcohol or drugs, they affect your moral reasoning and self-control. Have you lost the ability to determine what is right and what is wrong for you because you have used alcohol or drugs in the past? Do you need someone to force you to do the right thing, or are you capable of free will to do what you believe is the right thing? If you want to be responsible for yourself, you might want to contemplate the moral issues involved in continuing to drink or use drugs. Who is the best person to run your life?

Some people do not want the problems that getting drunk and high have caused them. They do not want to have to determine whether or not they have a problem with alcohol or drugs. They know the problems they have had from using alcohol or drugs. They just want to quit. They want to quit, so they will not have problems that result from drinking and drug use, like poor physical and mental health, legal issues, the financial cost, and the impact on their relationships. Other people want to quit because they don't want to get so loaded anymore. They became dissatisfied with how often they were using, how much they were using, or the height their intoxication was reaching. Many of those people discovered that when they wanted to quit, it was not easy to come up with reasons to make up their mind if they should quit forever or when they should quit forever. And, they didn't know when it is time to stop reasoning.

Have alcohol and drugs become so important to you that you can't even think about never getting loaded again? Are you thinking about a way to control the use of alcohol and drugs so that quitting forever will not be necessary? How you answer those questions will give you an indication of your values toward alcohol and drugs. Did you always feel that way about alcohol and/or drugs? Can you remember a time when they were not important to you? Think about the things you will not do without using alcohol and/or drugs. What is important to you? What do you want to do with your life and your time?

## Should You Go to Twelve-Step Groups Like AA and NA?

Before you go to any more twelve-step groups, read them verbatim:

## The Twelve Steps of AA:

Step 1:We admitted we were powerless over alcohol—that our lives had become unmanageable.

Step 2: We came to believe that a Power greater than ourselves could restore us to sanity.

Step 3: We made a decision to turn our will and our lives over to the care of God, as we understand him.

Step 4: We made a searching and fearless moral inventory of ourselves.

Step 5: We admitted to God, to ourselves, and to another human being the exact nature of our wrongs.

Step 6: We were entirely ready to have God remove all those defects of character.

Step 7: We humbly asked him to remove those shortcomings.

Step 8: We made a list of all the persons we had harmed, and became willing to make amends to them all.

Step 9: We made direct amends to such people wherever possible, except when to do so would injure them or others.

Step 10: We continue to take personal inventory and, when we were wrong, promptly admitted it.

Step 11: We sought through prayer and mediation to improve our conscious contact with God as we understand him, praying only for knowledge of his will and the power to carry that out.

Step 12: Having had a spiritual awakening as a result of these steps, we tried to carry this message to others and to practice these principles in all our affairs.

If after reading the steps you want to work them, go ahead and do that. Find a twelve-step group you can fit into. There are thousands of them. Please remember, I am not trying to talk anyone out of twelve-step attendance if you really want to go. I am pointing out facts about twelve-step attendance and logical contradictions with quitting forever. I am not knocking AA, NA, or any of the anonymous groups in total as organizations. I am holding them accountable for their teachings, but I am not trying to get them to change. They have been around since 1937 and have changed little. I do not want to change one word in AA's Twelve Steps or their literature..

Let's use critical thinking skills and examine the steps. Where in any of the Twelve Steps does it tell you how to keep from drinking or using? Which one even talks about not drinking or using? It sounds like faith healing or an old-time religion self-improvement program. It comes from the First-century Christian Fellowship started by Frank Buchman later know as the Oxford Group that started AA.

Did anyone ever tell you that the Twelve Steps were spiritual and not religious? That is deception. They have been found to be spiritual and religious under constitutional definition. The question is whether you believe you need religious activity in your life. If you do, why not return to the church, synagogue, mosque, or sweat lodge of your choice? Go to organized religion, or make up your own religion. Ask yourself if you should get involved with a group and engage in their religious activity while they deny it is religious activity.

If you are not religious, are agnostic, a secular humanist, or atheist, the *Big Book* of AA says your thinking is "soft and mushy," so you better give it up and believe them. They insult your nonbelief and tell you to give it up.

If you do believe, they are say your religious beliefs are not good enough to help you to abstain. You need to incorporate the above religious beliefs into your religion. Jews and Christians have told me their God commands they, "Have no other Gods before me." Twelve-step groups have told many that anything or anyone, including the group, can be your God. If your religious beliefs are offended by what they teach you in twelve-step groups, should you keep attending them?

I say your religion is good enough to help you abstain, and if you have no religious beliefs, you don't need to get them. Your time is better spent making up your mind whether you should ever again use alcohol or drugs. If you want to quit forever, that is what Quitting Forever is all about.

I have had some people come to me who wanted to continue attending AA and NA. Both people said it was like a social club. One person was the group secretary. Both liked helping to run the groups. Their only problem was they could not stay sober and away from drugs by attending twelve-step groups. They felt embarrassed every time they relapsed and got drunk or high again. They told me, "I don't want to give up the twelve steps. I just want to quit drinking and drugging." They both knew the twelve steps were religious activities and voluntarily wanted to participate.

I remind them the recovery groups were not always one day at a time. If you read the chapter "Working with Others" in the book *Alcoholics Anonymous* (3rd ed.), the advice is to "Ask him if he wants to quit for good and if he would go to any extreme to do so."

Both people quit forever quite rapidly. They no longer were afraid to be in places where alcohol or drugs were, because they made a decision to quit forever. Neither ever told the people in their twelve-step groups about quitting forever. They liked going to a group where they could make friends by calling themselves alcoholic and addict, saying how powerless they were, and working the twelve steps to run their lives. It was easier to work the steps once they discovered how to decide to end their alcohol and drug use by quitting forever.

## What is Twelve-Step Recovery and Relapse Prevention Like?

The recovery movement talks about the fact alcohol and drugs change your brain. They point out how the pleasure circuits hijack the prefrontal cortex part of the brain, where planning and decision making take place. Assume what they are saying is true, because there is a great deal of evidence to support this claim. Why do they keep the information of permanent exit from alcohol and drug abuse as an option for someone to consider? Instead of pointing out permanent abstinence is easily achieved by many and teaching how to carry it out, what is preached is twelve-step, one day at a time, and relapse prevention—what some call one urge at a time.

Review what the concept and experience of one-day-at-a-time recovery is like. The idea of one day at a time is that you say to yourself, "I promise I will not use for today, but I cannot and will not say I will not use tomorrow or anytime in the future, because I am an alcoholic/addict." Think about what the idea means. You have a task that is achievable. One of the things the concept of one day at a time is supposed to do is make your burden easier. Who wants to conceive of a lifetime without ever using alcohol and drugs again? After all, alcohol and drugs have hijacked your brain, so you will always have uncontrollable cravings for the stuff. How can you be expected to promise that you will never use it again? So, you play a trick on yourself. You only say you will not use for today. And, you carry it out day after day, going to support group meetings so they can support you in your not using one day at a time. Oh, by the way, you will be doing the twelve steps while you are getting support, and you will have to get a sponsor to tell you what to do and help you work the steps. Plus, you will have to find God, find a god, or make up your own god and start praying to it in a twelve-step fashion, all one day at a time. You have to admit you cannot do it without their help.

What is the experience of most people who attempt one day at a time? I say most, because 45 percent of people stop attending twelve-step groups in the first six months, and 95 percent have stopped within one year. One thing people have reported experiencing is realizing one day at a time means never drinking again if carried out for the remainder of their life. They say to themselves, "If I am going to carry out one day at a time for the remainder of my life, why am I doing it one day at a time? And, if I am doing it one day at a time, why do I have to never drink again for the remainder of my life?" Pondering the question leads to the twelve-step advice to stop pondering the question, because thinking about such a question is not carrying out one day at a time because you are thinking about the future. But, it is quite natural for humans to think about the future. People call it planning.

What is the experience of one-day-at-a-time recovery? Many people are very happy with one day at a time. It means they have the chance to drink again. They do not have to face the anxiety of never drinking again. The issue of whether they will drink again can remain unresolved. When an issue is resolved, you know how you think about it. But with one day at a time, you do not know how you will think about alcohol or drugs in the future. You can only get up and choose whether or not you are going to use alcohol or drugs for today. You have to choose either to do it or not do it. You have to deliberate. Deliberate means you have to think about using as well as not using. You have to pick one or the other to do for that day. You go to the twelve-step group to get support for making the choice not to drink or for disapproval, understanding, and forgiveness for drinking or using. A twelve-step group will help you accept the uncertainness of future drinking or drugging.

Other people are not happy with one-day-at-a-time recovery. They do not like the uncertainty of the future when it comes to drinking or drugs. Support and forgiveness seem demeaning to many who value self-reliance. "Why do I need support for not using or forgiveness and understanding if I use?" Not feeling supported and understood by a group can be an adverse experience. You came to the group to get help to prevent this from happening, and you were told to accept that there is no help other than from the supernatural as the result of doing the twelve steps. The most common report given to me is twelve-step group attendance makes you feel like drinking and using more, makes you feel depressed, or makes you feel angry.

There is nothing wrong with you if you have felt that way or currently feel that way now. You have freedom of conscience. You are the best one to decide what is right for you. You are not in denial. Wanting to avoid twelve-step groups is not a symptom of being an alcoholic or addict. The current rehabilitation wisdom is to not accept help that is not acceptable to you. You are the one to know best what is helping you.

## Relapse Prevention

Relapse prevention started out as an alternative to twelve-step recovery but has been absorbed by it. In relapse prevention, you learn to think differently about your drinking or drug use by learning to perform a hedonistic calculus where you weigh the reasons to drink against the reasons to abstain. By learning to think correctly when you recognize urges to drink, you figure out how to keep yourself from drinking each time an urge appears, one urge at a time. You are instructed to avoid places where alcohol is served and to watch for apparently irrelevant decisions, where you decide to go in a place where alcohol or drugs are present and eventually drink or use because of that. You have to learn and remember all your triggers. Relapse will happen unless you prevent it from happening.

Relapse is passive. It is a disease-model concept. For example, if you have pneumonia, you can get very sick and have to go to the doctor, who will give you antibiotic medication. Relapse occurs when you have taken all your medication and your pneumonia returns. Do you do anything to make it return? No. The pneumonia bacteria were still present in your lungs, and it multiplied all on its own. You did not have to do anything but just lie there. You relapsed into pneumonia.

Compare medical relapse to alcohol and drug relapse. There is not a trace of alcohol or drugs in your body. You reach out your hand, pick up alcohol or drugs, and put them in your body. You relapsed. Was that active or passive? Did it happen on its own, or did you make it happen? Why is it called relapse when it is something you did voluntarily?

It is often very difficult to think of reasons not to drink or drug when you want to. And, you have to lead your life like you are a second-class citizen. Other people can go places you cannot, because you have to prevent your relapse from happening. You better stay away from all places that sell alcohol or drugs, or you might make an apparently irrelevant decision.

Furthermore, you need support to do this. So, people were sent to twelve-step groups to get that support. AA and NA members have no difficulty with people from recovery treatment centers talking relapse prevention because one urge at a time fits nicely with one day at a time. With its high relapse rate, relapse prevention is no threat to AA or NA. And, it fits right into the model. You do the relapse prevention until you can call your twelve-step sponsor or get to a twelve-step group for the support you need. You can never be sure that you will never drink and/or drug again. You can practice relapse prevention while you work on getting through the twelve steps. Quitting forever is not an option.

Once you are in the twelve-step movement, you return and work the steps again and again, and do the relapse prevention for the remainder of your life. You live the twelve steps and make them your way of life. There is no way out. You are doomed to relapses of drunkenness and/or addiction if you leave the group.

Attending endless twelve-step groups and relapse prevention to stay clean and sober are not the only way. It is not even the way most people do it. Remember, AA acknowledged that 60 percent of the people who abstain do it without attending twelve-step groups. Most people do not think of themselves as alcoholics or addicts. They are confident about their ability to keep themselves from drinking/using in the future. There is a permanent exit for those who quit using forever. Once you realize you can keep yourself from using today, it is time to decide whether you will use ever again.

---

| Is relapse an active or passive event? |
| --- |

## People Underestimate Their Want to Drink Alcohol and Use Drugs

The feeling to drink or use drugs has been called irresistible. Brain studies show something physical happens when brain areas become excited. Physical brain reactions are really happening. What you experience is both physical and psychological. The physical reaction is your awareness of the brain excitement in response to some cue to drink or use a drug. The psychological reaction is the meaning you bring to the awareness of brain excitement. You have a response set to drink or use drugs that has been reinforced. People underestimate their reaction.

The physical reaction comes from the effects of using alcohol and drugs. Alcohol and drug use affect brain functions. Forebrain is your modern brain, called the cortex, which controls voluntary action. Alcohol and drugs change the way you think when you are under their influence. You think about things differently when you are loaded. But, alcohol and drugs also affect midbrain functions that control involuntary functions and emotions. Your midbrain controls involuntary reflexes and is where your pleasure pathways are located. The hindbrain control functions like heartbeat and respiration. When you use alcohol and drugs, you affect the pleasure pathways in the midbrain, and you feel pleasure. To some extent, it will override feelings of pain. It will also create a liking and a hunger for the substance which will make it seem more valuable to you. The physical reaction becomes conditioned to happen involuntarily in response to cues in the environment that become associated with the pleasure stimulated.

Stimulating the pleasure center in your brain feels good and is reinforcing. It reinforces your movements in consuming alcohol and/or drugs. Just repeating the act of consuming alcohol or drugs brings pleasure in what is called a response set. It becomes easy and even pleasurable to go through the motions of consuming your favorite substance. Once you start the response, it is hard to stop. The behavior competes with other possible behaviors that have been less reinforced. Your response set makes the action easy and pleasurable to do again.

Your psychological reaction is the determining part of the craving. It determines what you will do. Remember, alcohol and drug use changes your values while you are under the influence of alcohol or a drug and after you sober up or come down. The change is the increased value of importance for of alcohol or the drug you used. When you have a body reaction to a cue, you experience that importance of liking to use again. You remember the act of drinking or using a drug and how it made you feel good. Doing the act again and returning to the good feeling become more important with repeated use.

People often come up with reasons why they use, but most of the reasons probably came after they used, not before. We know people justify what they have done with reasons. Those justifications become reasons to use. That is why solving problems to keep you from using is an indirect and ineffective way to keep yourself from drinking and using drugs again. Solving problems gets you to go over your reasons to use. But, those were not really reasons to use, because they did not come before drinking or drugging; they came afterward. Going over your reasons to use can strengthen those reasons and make them more important to you. You will be chasing reasons and solving problems that might better be solved by not ever drinking or using.

With knowledge of what has happened to you and what is happening when you feel like drinking or using, the act of drinking or using a drug does not have to be irresistible. The feeling to use is not a cause to use but the result of using. Reasons to drink or use are justifications that likely came to you after you realized you drank or drugged and came up with explanations why you did it. People explaining why they did something are natural ways of thinking because we have been taught that we better have reasons for our actions. In reality, people do things without first having a lot of reasons; they come up with the reasons later.

Quitting forever means you will no longer use reasons to pick up alcohol or drugs and put them into your body. Quitting forever will not stop your body reactions. The body reactions are psychologically conditioned to occur as the result of your drinking and/or drugging. Those are the result of using alcohol or drugs and not the cause of your use. Body reactions will calm over time as the result of not using. You do not have to control them, because they are involuntary.

Quitting forever can change the psychological part of your reaction. Once you have decided you will never pick up alcohol or drugs again, it is time to become familiar with your physical and psychological reactions and accept them without trying to change them. Make room for them in your life. They are internal events from which you cannot run. You will control external events like controlling your hands instead of picking up alcohol or drugs to put into your body.

Recognizing you feel like drinking or using drugs tells you what you have done to yourself by drinking and/or drugging. It no longer needs to be a signal to drink or drug, because you do not pick it up; you are breaking the bonds of conditioning. Your response set is a tendency. You have other behaviors. Every time you feel like drinking or using and do not because of quitting forever, you are weakening your conditioned responses with one reason, quitting forever.

The value of alcohol and drugs changes after quitting forever. Observe your responses without running from them and without giving it any meaning other than awareness of actual thoughts and sensations. You do not call the thoughts or sensations good or bad. They are just there as evidence you drank alcohol and/or used drugs in the past. You will struggle if you try to push them away or suppress them, and they can become more intense. Accept them for what they are: just words in your head and body sensations and make peace with your response. If you try to shut them out of your experience, they may come back stronger. Make room in your experience for what alcohol and/or drugs have done to you but without consuming them again because of quitting forever. Alcohol and/or drugs are no longer important in your life. There are just the aftereffects.

You may think about drinking or using, but you do not have to buy the thought. When you buy a thought, you think about the thought and pursue it. Buying the thought and following where it takes you will always lead to the idea of drinking or using now or in the future. If you come up with a reason you should not to drink or use, there is always the corresponding reason of why you should drink or use. You can't have one without the other. Quitting forever means you no longer have reasons not to use or to use. There is just your experience of quitting forever. It is something you have done. It is more than a set of words you say to yourself; it is an internal experience that goes beyond words and is the value on which you act.

Just observe you are having the thoughts and feelings. If you are not going to pick up alcohol or drugs, they are nothing to fear. You cannot prevent the sensations, thoughts, and feelings from happening. They are automatic to some extent. Do not dwell on them or try to make them go away or you will be attempting to control them. If you try to keep them from happening, you create three problems for yourself:

1. You set up a rule that cannot be enforced. You are saying something should not happen that is likely to happen sometimes.

2. When you do feel like drinking and have the thoughts, it will feel like something is wrong like it shouldn't be occurring. You may feel surprised and anxious the thoughts and feelings are present. 3. You now have the problem of how to make them go away or control them. Or, you will have to find a way to ignore them by distracting yourself and pretending they do not exist, but you cannot fool yourself.

Saying you must not think about drinking or drugs after their repeated use is like falling into a hole and trying to dig yourself out. It seems like you are working hard to get out, but you are just digging yourself in deeper. Control your hands, and do not pick up alcohol or drugs because of quitting forever. You can control your external self. Do not try to control your inner self other than to observe it. What you are experiencing is partly an artifact of having a language, partly your thought history, and the rest is conditioning from drinking alcohol and/or using drugs.

Your thoughts and feelings only have to be controlled if quitting forever has not taken place. If not for quitting forever, you are delaying your use. Delaying use until later requires some control of thoughts and feelings. When you want to drink or use drugs and start thinking about it, other things that are going on can get in your way. But, if you have to wait to drink or use drugs, you have to focus your attention on those things that are getting in your way and making you wait to drink or use. You may have to wait until after work or until you can afford to drink or drug. You may have family and social activities that are getting in your way of drinking or drugging. You have to be able to control those feelings and thoughts to use so you can wait to do it.

Quitting forever ends the waiting to drink alcohol and use. You still have the physical and psychological feeling of wanting to use, but that feeling has a different value to you. You are not waiting to use. You are not battling the thoughts and feelings you know naturally result from your past. You are not worried they are present, because you are confident what you are going to do. You never drink alcohol or use drugs, so you are not waiting.

You willingly accept the thoughts and feelings and mindfully focus on what has to be done immediately. It is easy to figure out what is to be done, because drinking or using is eliminated from your consideration of choices. If you are at work, you focus on the task at hand. If you are with family or friends, you pay attention to them. When it is time to leave, you know you are not leaving to drink or use drugs because of quitting forever. Life takes on new meaning, because your values have changed now that alcohol and drugs are no longer important for you to consume.

# How important are alcohol and drugs to you?

## What Happened to You?

Alcohol and drugs changed your values. They changed your values when you were under the influence and when you sobered up. When you were under the influence of alcohol or drugs, you were disinhibited from doing things you would not do when sober. Disinhibited means your natural stops were numbed. Your moral code was lowered under the influence. When you sobered up and came off the alcohol or drugs, your values changed. The alcohol and drugs became more important. Alcohol and/or drugs keep becoming more important to you the more you return to getting high. Your brain chemistry was changed by drinking or drugging. It started to change back when you stopped.

People try alcohol or drugs for a variety of reasons. You aren't born using and didn't even know that there are alcohol or drugs to be consumed. As you grew older, you became aware that people were doing things to feel pleasure. Alcohol was part of our culture, and you saw stores selling it. You may have seen your parents or others drinking and/or drugging. At some point, you wanted to find out what it felt like.

Your first use was like an experiment. You didn't know what was going to happen, so you had to try the substance in the form of a personal experiment to find out how you would react. You didn't know what would happen if you drank alcohol or used a drug. You had the opportunity to drink or use a drug, and you made a choice to use or abstain. If you used and you found the experience pleasurable, perhaps you said to yourself on some level it was the thing to do. No immediate harm came to you. It felt good. Other people were doing it, and no harm seemed to come to them. Why not use it when you wanted to like others did? You likely made a decision to continue using. Your value about the substance you used was changed. You liked it better than before you used it. You changed your brain chemistry. You came up with reasons to do it again.

Once you knew what the substance felt like when you used it, you knew the pleasure it brought. Since you decided you would use the substance now and then, you used it now and then for fun, as recreational enjoyment. It was more fun to do things under the influence of alcohol or drugs. It made things feel more pleasurable. The substance either brought you up so you could party, or brought you down so you could relax. It was a thing to do with friends. Or, it became the thing to do when you were alone. Perhaps you started to use it to party and on other social occasions like holidays. Your values changed again, and drugs and/or alcohol became more important to your recreation and fun. You continued to change your brain chemistry, creating a conditioning reinforcement schedule.

With more experience using a substance, people start using it to help them get though demanding situations. A boring drive can be made more tolerable by having a few drinks, smoking some pot, or using some speed. If you didn't feel like doing something like mowing the lawn, using a substance made it easier. Visiting in-laws and talking with people you didn't like were easier to tolerate if you drank or used drugs. If life was boring, you were down or lonely, or if there was any situation you wanted to feel better about, you knew how to do it. Again, alcohol and/or drugs became more important, because you could depend on them to do something for you. Your brain was beginning to expect the reward of a chemistry change.

Many people learned something else about alcohol and drugs. You could use a larger amount quickly and really get a buzz. There was a stronger, more intense substance, like the difference between beer and distilled alcohol. You learned the difference between leaf and bud marijuana. You bought speed, coke, or heroin that was less stepped on and more pure. Sometimes you got more loaded than others and stayed that way for a longer time on a binge. And your values changed again, as alcohol and/or drugs could take you to another reality. Good, pure, or more potent stuff became more important. People who did not like to see you that high became less important. Your brain became accustomed to bigger rewards that lasted a longer time.

A relatively smaller number of people used alcohol and drugs so much and for long enough that they didn't feel right unless they were using. They became dependent on the substance to feel right. They felt very uncomfortable as the substance completely left their body. They used again to avoid that feeling and to feel like themselves, continuing the dependency. The dependency could be just psychological. It could be physical. Or, it could be both psychological and physical. Now, alcohol and/or drugs became really important. Keeping on the substance became very important because of what it felt like when you started to detox. Your brain accommodated to the presence of alcohol or a drug. Your brain chemistry was changed.

In all cases, using produced a pleasurable effect. The pleasure the substance produced and your increased value of the substance were the sole reasons for using. You formed a hunger for the substance. You fell in love with a certain buzz or high the substance produced, which was important for you to have again. Drinking or drug use created a desire to seek out that feeling again, because the substance became more important to you. No one tries to get addicted, and not everyone gets addicted, and not being addicted is no reason not to quit using. How much do you value alcohol and drugs over other things?

How important are alcohol and drugs to you? How much do you value them over other things? Importance is supported by reasons to keep drinking and drugging. Drinking alcohol or using drugs again tells how important they are to you no matter what you answer. What is important to you is determined more by what you do than what you think or say.

What happened to you was not a disease. What happened was the natural process of continuing to drink or use drugs the way you were. You might have tried to cut back, use less often, and go a long time without drinking or drugging. Cutting back was a reason to keep drinking and drugging. Drinking and drugging again after stopping for a period of time is more reinforcing behaviors; they strengthened the conditioning. Conditioning is not a disease. Conditioning is a natural process, the way your mind and body work together. Quitting Forever gives you the opportunity to put the conditioning in your hands.

You don't necessarily have to try to place yourself into any one of the above areas. They are not stages or categories. You don't have to try to determine if you are dependent or addicted or not. People move from one area to another, back and forth. One area does not necessarily lead to the next. What happens is that people try to balance their use to get the benefits and avoid the costs of using. People who are using are really trying to get the pleasure and avoid the pain of what happens when they use. They are not focused on some of the problems alcohol or drugs have caused and do not want to talk about it. That is perception and not denial.

Helpers may call you an alcoholic or addict. When you said you are not they yelled, "denial." Maybe you were then confronted with how much you use and some of the problems you don't want to talk about. In that case, you are not in denial but in disagreement with your accuser, since alcoholic and addict are not diagnoses but demeaning labels that one naturally wants to avoid.

Not everyone avoided the label of alcoholic or addict. Some people took the label and identified with it. Alcoholic or addict became an identity or self-concept. A verbal convention became a reality trap because of words and the use of language. They looked at themselves from the perspective of the label and explained their drinking and drug use on that basis. The label of alcoholic or addict became another reason to keep using the substance.

Other people will try to convince you that you have a problem with alcohol or drugs to give you a reason to quit. You may or may not have a problem with alcohol and drugs, but if you do, you already know it. Having a problem with alcohol or drugs is certainly a reason to quit using them forever, but not having a problem with alcohol or drugs is no reason for not quitting forever. You are not in denial when you do not want to call yourself alcoholic or addict. You are disagreeing with the person who is telling you about your problem for a variety of reasons. Your arguing to continue your use of alcohol or drugs lets you know how important and valuable they have become to you. How have your values changed to become more positive toward using drugs and/or drinking alcohol? If alcohol and drugs seem part of who you are, you may have avoided the label but are still trapped by language. You may be lost in thought, where your reasons to drink alcohol or use drugs are more important than your experience of using them.

What makes alcohol or drugs so important to you? What are you willing to give up to continue using drugs or to drink alcohol? Whatever you are willing to give up to keep using alcohol and/ or drugs can tell you something. Drugs and/or alcohol have become more important to you than whatever you are willing to give up. Even if you are going to do something less often or not as long, alcohol and/or drug use is competing for your time and energy. You may not be reacting to the overall affect of your alcohol or drug use; you may be reacting to your ideas about using alcohol and drugs. Those ideas are some of your reasons to keep using. Those reasons support your values of using alcohol or drugs.

Whether or not you have a problem with alcohol or drugs, drinking alcohol or using drugs may have caused you a problem or problems. What follows is a list of yes and no questions followed by questions for you to rate on a scale of 1 to 7 to help you review your experience about some of the problems drinking alcohol or using drugs might have caused you.

## Self-Analysis Survey

| | | | |
|---|---|---|---|
| Have alcohol or drugs caused any problems you wished never happened? | | Yes | No |
| Did you sometimes feel like getting extremely drunk or high? | | Yes | No |
| When drunk or high, have you ever said something you wished not said? | | Yes | No |
| Has anyone ever had advantage over you because you were drunk or high? | | Yes | No |
| Did you ever avoid someone because you were drunk or high? | | Yes | No |
| Were you ever unable to sleep because you were drunk or high? | | Yes | No |
| Did you ever go to work under the influence of alcohol or drugs? | | Yes | No |
| Did you ever go to work hung-over or coming down off a drug? | | Yes | No |
| Did you ever have a problem at work related to drinking or drugs? | | Yes | No |
| Did you ever drive under the influence of alcohol or drugs? | | Yes | No |
| Have you had any legal problems related to alcohol or drugs? | | Yes | No |
| Have you ever spent more money than you wished on alcohol or drugs? | | Yes | No |
| Have you ever sold drugs to buy drugs? | Yes | No | N/A |
| Have you ever sold or pawned anything to buy alcohol or drugs? | | Yes | No |
| Did you ever do anything you were ashamed of while drunk or high? | | Yes | No |
| Did you ever say you would not drink or drug and do it anyway? | | Yes | No |
| Has alcohol or drugs caused you other problems you can acknowledge? | | Yes | No |

If yes, then list some of the other problems drinking or drugging has caused you:

How important is your drinking and/or your drug use to you?

| | Not | 1 | 2 | 3 | 4 | 5 | 6 | 7 | Very |

How addicted do you think you were to alcohol or drugs?

| | None | 1 | 2 | 3 | 4 | 5 | 6 | 7 | Totally |

How addicted do you think you are now to alcohol or drugs?

| | None | 1 | 2 | 3 | 4 | 5 | 6 | 7 | Totally |

How much do you want to return to controlled use of alcohol or drugs?

| | None | 1 | 2 | 3 | 4 | 5 | 6 | 7 | Totally |

Can you think of the idea or envision yourself never using alcohol or drugs again?

| | Cannot | 1 | 2 | 3 | 4 | 5 | 6 | 7 | Vision |

How much effort are you willing to put into quitting alcohol or drugs?

| | None | 1 | 2 | 3 | 4 | 5 | 6 | 7 | Highly Motivated |

How ready are you to take action to quit alcohol and drugs forever?

| | Never | 1 | 2 | 3 | 4 | 5 | 6 | 7 | As Soon as Possible |

Rate your ability for quitting alcohol or drugs forever.

| | Can't | 1 | 2 | 3 | 4 | 5 | 6 | 7 | Able |

Rate your doubt about being able to carry out quitting forever.

| | No doubt | 1 | 2 | 3 | 4 | 5 | 6 | 7 | Un-doable |

## You Can't Convince Yourself to Quit Forever

Follow Your Values and Decide

Convincing generally occurs when one person talks to another person and sells them on an idea. When someone is trying to convince you to do something, that is their purpose or what they have set out to do. Deliberation is a form of reasoning, when you are figuring out what to do. Once you have figured it out, then you know what to do. When you are trying to convince yourself, your purpose is to persuade yourself into a belief. That may not work well. You cannot convince yourself to abstain by saying to yourself a thousand times, "I will never again drink alcohol or use drugs." That will not work, because you will hear words in your head saying you will drink or use drugs again.

People who make up their mind do not have to persuade themselves to want something to happen. Sometimes, people who want something to happen persuade themselves to take action to get something to happen. But, doing some action because you want something to happen is different than thinking something to generate the want. You may not like what you are doing to make something happen, but you are pleased when it happens, because the outcome is important to you. It seems like the thing to do, because it is important to you. You do not have to persuade yourself to think only of the thing that seems as though it should be done. Thoughts about doing something will be in your mind even if you are not going to do it. Do you want to drink or use drugs again? What are your values about continuing use? Are you stuck in your reasoning? You may be experiencing ambivalence.

# Ambivalence About Quitting Forever

The arrow illusion is an example of the experience of ambivalence. You can see arrows pointing one way. Can you see them pointing the other way? On one hand, you would like to not have problems caused by drinking and drugs, but on the other hand, you do not want to give up the wonderful high alcohol and drugs give you. You think about quitting, but you switch back to thinking about using. You feel like you never want to use again, then you feel like using. Part of what you are experiencing is perceptual. There is no point of reference to anchor your mind. The arrows don't switch back and forth, but your mind sees it that way. If you follow your mind, you

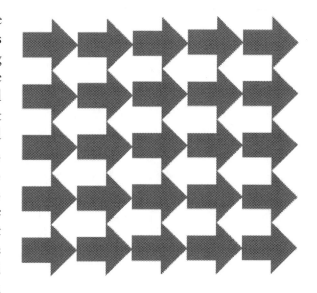

will always be switching back and forth. You can choose to see the arrows pointing one way, but you will have to keep choosing, because you will see them pointing the other way. Either your mind will see the arrows switch back and forth, or you will keep choosing which way to follow.

What is ambivalence? Look it up in the dictionary; ambivalence is not one of the words made up by the recovery movement. Basically, ambivalence is when you are attracted and repelled by the same thing. It is approach-avoidance conflict. You can't do both, so thinking about one makes you think about doing the other, and your mind is not set on which one to do. You go back and forth between two mutually exclusive ideas, undecided about which one you will do. Mutually exclusive means that if you do one, you cannot do the other; you cannot do both. You are undecided on which one to do. You may choose one for a while, but the other is always open for the choosing. The choice keeps returning.

Look at the arrow illusion. You can make up your mind which direction you will follow. The arrows do not have to stop pointing back and forth for you to make up your mind on which direction you follow. What do you use as your point of reference to know which way to decide?

What does your experience tell you? You have your values, but drinking alcohol or using a drug has affected them.

## Exercise

1. What has happened before as the result of my drinking or using drugs?

Immediate results:

Short-term results:

Long-term results:

2. Draw a timeline of your life showing when you were using and what followed.

3. What would you advise someone to do about drinking or using drugs again if they had the history you wrote down above?

4. What are the risks of an undesirable outcome continuing?

5. Are you willing to accept the undesirable outcome? How would you feel? What would you be doing? Are you following your values?

6. You had a bad outcome before from using alcohol and/or drugs. Are you willing to risk it happening again? Why is it so important for you to take that risk?

7. Think about what to do about your use of alcohol and/or drugs again, and what you should do. Why is this important? How does drinking/using compete with other things important to you?

## When Making up Your Mind Weigh Both Sides

One side will seem more favorable. If you have to convince yourself, you may be arbitrarily picking one side and then saying that is what you will do without addressing the other side enough. You can address your ambivalence, the positive and negative of both sides. You may be weighing consequences and going back and forth. The question is what will this thought do for me? not what does it mean to me?

Ask yourself, what will happen as the result of my drinking and/or drugging? What has happened before? Would you advise someone else to do that? Is it without risk of a bad thing happening? Are you willing to accept that bad thing if it happened? Will it be so bad if it happened again? Are you willing to stand it if it happens again? What do you want to have happen in terms of your use of alcohol or drugs again? Do you have a clear value to follow?

If you feel regret about not quitting forever sooner, you have a signal that reflects your actual experience. What could you have done if you weren't drinking and/or drugging the way you were this last year? Where would your life be now if you were never drinking or drugging some time ago?

## People just look for reasons to not drink.

Relapse prevention gets makes you come up with lots of reasons not to drink to convince yourself not to drink or use in the face of an urge to drink or use. With twelve step, one day at a time, you convince yourself not to drink or use just for today. Both ways, you have to keep re-convincing yourself. That leaves room for error if you can't re-convince yourself. If you have to re-convince yourself, you have not resolved your ambivalence about drinking and using. And, it keeps you thinking about drinking or using. You cannot think about not using without thinking about using. They go together like heads and tails.

When you look at the reasons why you want to drink again, you better understand the brain model of recovery. Without understanding the brain model of recovery, you will be addressing problems as though they make you want to drink, and you will be led back to solving problems to keep from drinking. Basically, the part of your brain that was hijacked to want and think about alcohol and/or drugs does not control the part of your brain that voluntarily lets you move your hands. Why? There are no nerves directly connecting the two brain areas. Your hands are not hard-wired with nerves to the part of your brain calling out for alcohol or drugs. Wanting and using come from two different brain areas. Wanting cannot make using happen unless you voluntarily move your hands to make it happen. Liking it and wanting to use it again are two different parts of your brain.

## The Real Reason You Want to Use Alcohol and/or Drugs

The reason you want to pick up drink or drugs is the good way they make you feel when you use them, not because your problems make you feel bad. You are not running from problems but toward intoxication. Reexamine the reasons you want to return to that feeling of being drunk or high. Those are words in your head. What does your experience tell you? If you are thinking about running from your problems, remember that is recovery industry talk and will not lead you to a solution about whether to quit alcohol or drugs. It will lead you to problem solving of those problems. Personal problem solving is an indirect and defensive approach when you solve a personal problem to prevent a relapse. You will feel like using again when you have problems again and when you have no problems.

Think of it this way. If your problem was solved and you were not feeling upset, you would only be feeling neutral. Would that be good enough for you to not want to drink or use drugs? The answer is likely no, it would not be enough. Feeling neutral is not feeling drunk or high on drugs. And, now you could either say to yourself, "What is the harm of getting loaded because I don't have any problems." Or, you might think of celebrating. "I solved my problem. Things are better. Let me celebrate my success by using." You know you are feeling good, and you know how much better you could feel.

## Listen to Your Mind Plead and Bargain for Alcohol and/or Drugs

Now, separate from that voice and just observe what is going on. Understand it for what it is. The voice is words in your head. What is it trying to get you to do? Is that something you want to do again, or are you being persuaded by it? Listen to those ideas for what they are: drinking or using drugs. Ask yourself, "Are those my ideas to use, or are they words in my head?" If you want to end the problem and stop using, then any idea to drink or use drugs is your mind chattering words. You do not have to accept ideas to drink or use as your ideas anymore. You just accept them as just words in your brain. There is a difference between having an idea and buying into the idea. People get caught up in avoiding or controlling their internal state. One of the ways you separate from the brain words of addiction is to treat them as a separate idea of words, feelings, and sensations. Just observe and describe them. Learn how to observe your internal state without giving it any value or buying into it. You do not have to control your inner state of mind once you know what you are going to do. You control your external state.

You control your external state by controlling your hands. Will drinking or drugging ever become a good idea again? Do you want to drink again or not? If you are not going to drink again, then why does your internal state have to be controlled? Until you come to accept that you are going to have thoughts and feeling to use again, you are going to see them as reasons to do so. Once you can experience them as an internal state that does not control you, you can act on your values of what is really important to you. Make room for those thoughts. They are just words and sensations. They do not directly cause you to move your hands.

## Exercise

Say to yourself, like whispering words in your head, "Stand up," but do not stand up. Don't do it. Say the words again, and just sit there. Did the words in your mind cause you to stand up when you thought them, or were they just words in your mind?

Write down any idea about drinking or using drugs that pops into your mind. Any idea that has alcohol or drugs is recognized and written. The thought could be about the past, present, or future. The idea doesn't have to be directly about using. It may be a memory of how good it was to use, how you might be able to get away with it and do it again someday, or doubts about not being able to go without alcohol or drugs. Write anything that has to do with your drinking or using drugs that comes to your mind, either when you are trying to think about it or when you are not trying to think about it.

If you do not want to drink or use drugs again, any ideas about alcohol or drugs are just words passing through your mind. Come to recognize them as just words or ideas passing through your mind. The words are not actually alcohol and drugs coming at you. You do not have to stop them, change them, or control them. It will always lead you back to drinking or using drugs again if you buy into them. Just observe and describe them. They are like signs along the side of the road you go by on the highway. You observe yourself seeing them but you have no intention on stopping to follow them. They are just there.

Relax and focus your eyes on something or close. Observe the thoughts and feelings inside you without giving them value or catching onto them. Let any thought about alcohol or drugs pass through your mind the same way. Talk about your experience with this exercise.

Are you still going to use alcohol or drugs again? How do you feel toward a set of ideas that is trying to get you to do something you think should not be done? It is a day of decision. You can decide if you will ever use alcohol or drugs again. Why would you put off the decision?

Once you can recognize those ideas, and you don't want to drink and/or drug again, you don't have to argue against them. If you have made your decision never to drink or drug, you no longer value the ideas to drink or use. They do not control you, because you do not try to control them. Make up your mind. Will you drink or use drugs again? You have to pick one side or the other, or your ambivalence will remain. No one can make up your mind for you. What do you want to do with your life? What is important to you? Those are your values. Will the thoughts about drinking alcohol or using drugs help you do what you want to do with your life?

Once your mind is made up, you have determined what to do. Once your mind is decided you made an action decision. You have a value to follow. If you hear ideas to drink or use, do not buy into them. Making up your mind does not mean stopping the thoughts to drink or use drugs from passing through your mind. Making up you mind means you have decided what actions you are going to do.

Make up you mind, and stop re-figuring out what to do. Once you know about how your mind works, you know your mind is not you because you made a decision. You don't have to accept those ideas as yours. Accept the words and sensations as being present when you are aware of them. Words going back on your decision are coming from the other part of your brain. Treat them like they are: words passing through. Do not act like you are talking to yourself. You know what is happening, and you do not have to control your inner words if you do not value them. Now, you are not trying to convince yourself you will never drink again. It is something you make happen. Make it happen by acting on it. You decided to make it happen, and now you are carrying out your decision.

## Hold onto Your Decision to Never Drink or Drug Again

You don't have to make the thoughts of drinking or using go away. You just have to know what you are going to do when you hear or feel them, and you have to know the words in your head do not control your hands. Your mind will try to get you to solve problems to keep yourself from drinking. What a deal. As soon as you can't solve a problem, then it is time to drink or drug. Part of making up your mind is deciding that you will never drink or use drugs again, even if you have problems. Solve problems to get a solution to the problem and not to keep yourself from drinking or drugging.

---

## You do not have to run from thoughts and feelings

## Do you feel any doubt about carrying out your decision?

Doubt is the part of the natural process of quitting forever. Recognize your doubt and give it voice. Does that doubt help you follow your values of never drinking or drugging? Will that doubt help you carry out your decision? Your doubts are reasons to use drugs or drink alcohol. It is not what your doubt says to you, but what it will do for you.

If you doubt your ability to abstain, it is time to read the brain-recovery model. If you doubt your decision, recognize that doubt by writing it on paper. Read what you have written. Say it one hundred times. Does it have any real meaning to you? Is your mind less made up now that you are reading about your doubt than when you made your decision to never drink or use drugs again? Do you still never want to use alcohol and drugs again? Face the doubt. Make up your mind in the face of doubt. You know what to do. You do not have to persuade or convince yourself what to do. You can recover and end this problem anytime you want. Do you want to end it or try another round of drinking and drugs? You are going to have to face that decision and hold it or start deliberating and choosing. What do you want to have happen? How many times do you want to go back and re-figure it? You can end the struggle with a decision you act on. Who controls your hands? Recovery is in your hands. Look at your hands. What will you do with them? If you do not know, you have not made up your mind to make a decision.

# Recovery is in your hands

## Your Mind is Not Made Up, and You Feel Like a Drink/Drug

Maybe you will never feel like drinking or using drugs again. But don't bet on it. It is more than likely you will feel like drinking or using drugs again. If you are not prepared, you will not know what to do. You will have to figure out what to do at the worst time. The worst time to figure out if you should drink alcohol or use drugs is when you feel like drinking or using drugs.

When you feel like having a drink or using a drug and you do not know what you will do ahead of time, you will look for cues. You will look for internal cues and external cues. Internal cues are thoughts that cross your mind, sensations you are aware of, and feelings you have. External cues are things you see, hear, taste, and smell. With the right internal and external cues in place, you will drink alcohol or use drugs again, or try them for the first time if you have not used. Sometimes internal cues come to awareness first. Sometimes external cues come to awareness first.

Some examples of external cues coming to awareness first are when you are around other people who are drinking or using. You go out with friends or a loved one. They are drinking and having a good time. You order dinner, and your partner orders a favorite beverage. The server asks you what you would like. You are offered free alcohol or drugs. Someone offers you a good deal to buy your favorite drug very cheap. You are offered a rare chance to use a very pure or high-potency dose of your favorite drug or alcoholic beverage. You are offered a drug or drink you have never tried, and you are curious.

Some examples of internal cues can be feeling like getting a little high on alcohol or drugs, feeling like using a little bit; wishing you were loaded, having a good time like everyone else; feeling uncomfortable you are not high; and feeling excited about the prospect of drinking or using a drug, and then feeling frustrated as you wait and do not use. Some people feel angry they cannot drink or use drugs. Other people feel lonely when they want to drink or use. People have told me they felt happy or sad or bored, and it made them want to use.

## Exercise

Write it down.

What is your valued plan for when you feel like drinking or drugging again?

Complete either a., b., or c.

a. It is important I drink and/or drug again because …

b. I can't make up my mind what is the right thing for me to do because …

c. It is important in never drink or use drugs again because …

# Quitting Forever: The Basics

Hopefully, you are reading this because you want to find out about how to quit alcohol and drugs forever.

Make sure you are not under the influence of alcohol or drugs when you think about quitting forever. If it is too difficult for you to stop, go to a detox center until you have withdrawn from the effects of alcohol or drugs. The only risk in using a detox center is many will push the disease concept and preach the twelve steps. Bring them this book and have them call me. I will be happy to assist you in planning your detox with them.

Remember, when people make an organized plan, it can be difficult to change the plan.

Here are some basic explicit instructions on Quitting Forever. What is talked about here is reiterated and expanded further in more depth in the "Natural Process of Quitting Forever."

1. The first place to begin is to admit to yourself no one can do this but you. Ask yourself, "Do I really want to do this forever? Really?" No one can really help you quit forever or carry it out. It is something you will have to do on your own. Quitting is not a group activity. You will have to do it alone and privately. You will often have to carry it out when you are alone and sometimes against the encouragement of others to drink or drug. You can talk about it with other people quitting forever.

2. You do not have to have good reasons to quit. But, they better be your own reasons, not anyone else's. Someone else's reasons to quit really won't matter that much to you. But, get ready to go beyond reasons, because if reasons continue to matter, you can't say that you quit forever and reasons to drink or drug no longer matter. What are your values? What is important to you?

3. After quitting forever, stop using reasons why you won't drink or drug again. Once you quit, you only have one reason you will do not drink or use drugs. That reason is because of quitting forever, and now you never drink alcohol or use drugs. If you are still listening to reasons, then you are bargaining, not carrying out what you have done. If you are reasoning, bargaining, or counting time, those are not part of quitting forever. Quitting Forever means only one reason, and you no longer question that reason. You do not try to control your mind to keep you from thinking about using. You have a value to act on. You make a decision and stop choosing. Words to drink or drug have no meaning.

4. Make sure that you know you can carry out your decision, self-pledge, promise, or plan. If you have any doubts about your ability, then you can't give yourself a 100 percent promise. Quitting Forever is a promise with no doubts that you will carry it out in the face of feeling like drinking or using. You will no longer run from being in the presence of alcohol or drugs, because that is your chance to act on your value to never drink or drug. You seek out chances to feel like drinking and drugging and to carry out your plan and ability to abstain until the task becomes meaningless to you. You are good at what you do and know that you will always carry it out. That can't happen if you have doubts or feel unsure about your ability. Find a way to get really sure you can do this. You have to get past the disease concept to carry it out. You have to know why drinking and drugging is always voluntary or you may have doubts.

5. Pick a date and time to carry out quitting forever. If it is in the future and something that you want to do, bring it to a present date and time. Say to yourself, "Now I am quitting forever and after this time I no longer drink alcohol or use drugs for any reason." Now that you have said it, check to see if you have any doubts that you will do it. Do you not want to follow the value you just said to yourself? It is not too late. If you are not going to follow your value, then say to yourself, "I quit forever, and I will never change my mind about that no matter what the reason or for how long." Now, it is done. You have set something up that has to be changed before you can drink or drug. If you are religious or spiritual, you can strengthen your pledge by promising your God or gods that you will never drink or drug again. A promise to yourself is sufficient, and if you are religious, it has to start with a promise to yourself. Remember the saying, "God helps those who help themselves." Now that it is done, how do you feel? Quitting forever is your guiding value.

6. Address your doubts about carrying it out by returning to your pledge or plan. Address doubts about your ability by returning to your understanding of how your brain and body work together biologically. Part of what you have done is a made a decision. The other part of what you do is having the experience of carrying out the decision.

7. Imagine alcohol and drugs right in front of you. Look at them and feel like drinking and using. As soon as you recognize that feeling to drink or use, think, *I do not have to control this or make it go away, because I never drink or drug.* Accept any feeling and thoughts to use as just passing by. Do not struggle with them. Let them be. Make room for them in your experience.

They were caused by using and are not commands to drink or use. Get ready to use that skill when you feel like using or when alcohol or drugs are present.

Be mindful of thoughts and feelings to use without buying into them. Observe them as just thoughts and feelings. They are words and sensations and not guiding principles or values. Imagine the words in your head as autumn leaves falling across a blue sky. Watch them drift down into a babbling brook to be carried away. Do not give those thoughts value or meaning. They're just words passing by. Let them be meaningless chatter in your mind.

Go on and live your life like you want. Do whatever you want to do. Go wherever you want to go. You are no longer addicted unless you use again. You may become more detoxed, but you cannot become more recovered than never using alcohol and drugs. You don't change yourself to keep from using alcohol or drugs. You quit alcohol or drugs and change your life to fit just you and your image of someone who never drinks alcohol or uses drugs. Your days of living the life of a second-class citizen are over. You are back to being like everyone else who doesn't drink or use drugs. You can go anywhere you want and do what you want, because under no circumstances are you ever going to drink alcohol or use drugs.

Every time you get the thought or feeling to use, you recognize that feeling for what it is. It is an internal state. It is another part of you making words and feelings. Do not struggle with it. It does not control your hands to pick up alcohol and drugs. Just recognize and observe the words and sensations in your body. Do not give them meaning with more words.

# Question the Brain-Disease Concept

Quitting forever cannot happen if you think you have a disease that makes you pick up alcohol or drugs when you do not want to. Since the recovery helpers still talk about addiction as a brain disease, let me give you a dose of the brain-disease concept model to scrutinize. Do you believe everything someone in authority tells you? Disease is not a concept. Disease is a fact. When the American Medical Association classified addiction as a disease, they voted to make it so. They do not vote to classify real diseases. The evidence is there for real diseases, and there is no need to vote. Examine the concepts closely, and determine for yourself if you can find contradictions. I will explain why it seems like a disease to some people.

## Infectious-Disease Concept

Which seems more plausible to you? Start out understanding why they say alcohol and drug addiction are like infectious diseases, and then read the rational critical response. Pick the concept that seems the most reasonable to you.

Alcohol and drug addiction are like infectious diseases. In an infectious disease, a virus or bacteria infects some people but not everyone. There are different degrees of immunity based on a complex set of genetic and environmental factors. They include your genetics, ethnicity, degree of crowding, and status of your immune system. Certainly, people carrying an infectious disease give it to uninfected people. So, people who are not infected get it from people who are infected.

Infectious disease is spread best by people who have caught it. And so it is with alcohol and drug addiction.

In alcohol and drug addiction, users primarily transmit new behaviors to their peers. Like an infection, addiction is spread easier in populations where there is more crowding. Some ethnic groups are more susceptible to a disease than other ethnic groups. Some people are more immune to addiction than other people because of their genetic makeup. In that way, alcohol and drug addition is like an infectious disease.

However, if you think critically, and I hope you will, you will see that alcohol and drug addiction are not like infectious diseases at all. No bacteria or virus enters your body. To say that alcohol and drugs are like living organisms is like using ancient thoughts of animism. Animism is when people attributed life to inanimate objects. There is lack of scientific bases for that notion.

Alcohol and drugs enter your body because you consciously put them there. Viruses and bacteria are unseen and enter your body through the air or on some food or beverage you eat or drink. You do not consume to get virus and bacteria, but you do consume to get alcohol and drugs into your body. You purposely put alcohol and drugs in your body for the effects. Furthermore, when virus and bacteria enter your body, they reproduce and become more. You are sicker the next day even if you did not put anymore of the microorganisms in your body. Alcohol and drugs don't reproduce in your body. The substances become less once they enter your body because they are metabolized. You have less in you the next day, and if you do not use more, it will completely leave your body. Your brain chemistry is changed, but it changes back to normal as the result of not drinking or using drugs.

You are not susceptible to alcohol and drugs. You are susceptible to the idea of using them. It is not the alcohol and drugs but the idea of getting high and having fun that you want to use. Are ideas like virus and bacteria also? This is getting ridiculous.

And, if you do put alcohol and/or drugs into your body, you can stop anytime. With bacteria and viruses, you cannot stop. You have to get antibiotics to treat the bacteria or other medications to treat the virus, or wait until your body builds immunity to the microorganisms. With viruses and bacteria, you have no choice. With alcohol and/or drugs, you do have a choice. You cannot decide never to get a cold again, but you can decide to never drink or drug again. Many people of all ages, ethnicities, genetic makeup, and who live under good or poor conditions are quitting forever after they have used alcohol and/or drugs.

> ## You can't quit a disease that makes you drink or use drugs.

## Compulsive-Obsession Disease Concept

Alan Leshner, Director of the National Institute on Drug Abuse (NIDA), talks about the disease model of addiction. The brain disease starts out with voluntary behavior that ends in "uncontrollable compulsive drug craving." I question the uncontrollable and compulsive statement. Uncontrollable means incapable of being controlled. But, how many drug users are using out in public? They are able to control their use enough to keep it hidden. We have to use drug testing and special agents to catch drug users, because they keep so much control over their drug use that the general public does not see it. They control their use but not to our standards of control; so, we say they have lost control. Furthermore, the majority of those addicted have gone through treatment and started using again after detox, when they were not out of control because they were drunk or high from alcohol or drug use.

Compulsion is a behavior that has to be carried out. Alcohol and drug users don't have to drink and use. Nothing forces you to drink or drug when you do not want. You voluntarily move you arms and hands to pick it up and consume the drink or drug.

Some may have an obsession about using, meaning they have a persistent preoccupation to use. But, the individual faced with the task of quitting is the one best to determine how obsessed he or she is. Obsession means thoughts of alcohol or drugs just pops into your mind and doesn't go away. Obsession is only at the extreme. Most people who use alcohol and drugs fall between volitional thought and an obsessed thought. You do not have to buy into obsessive thoughts.

When does the voluntary use become truly involuntary? Be careful here, because this is where we give the user an excuse for what they are doing, when we could help them see what they are doing is voluntary.

## Biological-Disease Concept

Alcohol and drug addiction are likened to diabetes and high blood pressure. You may or may not have done things to bring on the chronic disease, but once it is there, you have to manage it. The symptoms will go away, but you will always have the disease. The problem with this concept is that diabetes and high blood pressure is the person's natural state. That is their body condition at rest if they do nothing to prevent it. Someone with diabetes has an insulin problem because of his or her pancreas. They either have low or high blood sugar.

Someone with an alcohol problem has high alcohol content. But, at rest when sober, they have no alcohol in their bloodstream, and neither does the person addicted to drugs test positive for drug use. His or her body condition at rest is clean and sober, unless they do something to change that. It is completely the opposite from the person with diabetes. Remember, we diagnose the problem by the presence of high blood alcohol content or a positive drug test. The person with diabetes has to do something to prevent the problem. The alcoholic or addict has to do something to make intoxication happen.

Let's illustrate it again with a simple comparison experiment. Since the person with diabetes and the person with an alcohol/drug problem have similar type diseases, then let's sit them down together and watch for symptoms. Imagine it is 8:00 in the morning, and we start the experiment in a room that neither the diabetic nor alcoholic/addict can leave. They have nothing to keep them occupied; and they just have to sit. Now, it is noontime. Observe the diabetic feeling weak and ill. The alcoholic/addict is not feeling too well either, but was detoxed. Measure the diabetic's blood sugar level, and it is going up due to low insulin. Measure the alcoholic's blood alcohol level, and it is still zero. An addict tests negative for the presence of drugs. Now, it is going into the afternoon.

The diabetic smells fruity because of low insulin and acts like a drunk. The alcoholic/addict is still clean and sober and has a blood alcohol level of zero or a negative drug test. If we continue the experiment for a few days, the diabetic will become sick and die, while the alcoholic/addict will become healthier.

How can these be similar diseases? They cannot, because the alcoholic/addict did not have a real disease. Alcoholic and addict is an identity not a disease. I think we insult people with real diseases by calling alcohol and drug addiction a disease. Can you imagine giving a diabetic the chance to quit his or her disease?

## A Disease or a Natural Aftereffect of Drinking or Using Drugs

You do not have a disease preventing you from quitting forever. You have affected your brain and behavior. You affected your brain when you used alcohol or a drug. Brain chemistry change is what makes you feel high. The brain chemistry change has an aftereffect. The brain chemistry change aftereffect is reinforcement you can feel and recognize. Your involuntary nervous system was affected, and your voluntary nervous system was affected. The problem with the disease concept is using this information to show you there is no way out. You are permanently marked. With the brain-recovery model, you use this information as a way out of continued alcohol and drug use. You are freed.

Brain chemistry is why you feel pleasure. It is natural to feel pleasure in response to things like food, water, and sex. It has survival value for humans as a species. When you feel good after eating, drinking water, or having sex, your dopamine levels rise in a part of your brain called the nucleus accumbens, which is found in your midbrain. As the result of genetics and conditioning, it works both ways. Your brain alerts you to the presence of food, water, and sex so you can consume it and stay alive or reproduce. Rewards of consuming reinforce you to consume again. Rewards can help you adapt to your environment. Rewards tell you what is valuable to you.

Alcohol and drugs are reinforcing in the same way. However, they can compete with your attention and thoughts, because they can become increasingly reinforcing. This means you like them more. A part of your brain says, "I want more of that." Thoughts of drinking or drugging pop into your mind without trying. That part of your brain is a primitive part, the old brain. It is a part of your brain that is involuntary to orient you to things in your environment to keep you alive and reproduce by giving you a pleasure reward when you do it. But, alcohol and drugs can override other things that are rewarding in three ways: (1) competing for your attention and thoughts, (2) producing more pleasure by acting directly on pleasure centers, and (3) becoming more important and valuable to you.

How would you know how much this has happened to you? Think about how much you like to drink or use your favorite drug. If you like it—or really like it—you can feel what was just described. If you think about alcohol or drugs without really trying, you know it is competing for your thoughts. Does the thought of drinking alcohol or using a drug stick in your mind? If it is easy for you to notice other people who are drinking or using drugs, it is competing for your attention. If it is easy to notice when alcohol or drugs are present, it is competing for your attention.

You might notice some body sensations like excitement or nervousness when you have thoughts about drinking or using drugs. Those are natural feelings most people have sometimes when they anticipate getting something they want. It may feel uncomfortable not to move toward and pick up alcohol or drugs when they are around. It may feel as though you are depriving yourself. Your heart may beat faster. Your attention may narrow in focus, noticing where alcohol and/or drugs are found. It is possible to feel alarmed. It may be difficult to look away or go on like you had not noticed other people using or that alcohol and drugs were present. You may feel like talking about drinking or drug use. Images of past good times using may cross your mind.

You might want to talk to someone you drank or used drugs with about how you did it together. If you are with strangers, you may feel left out and alienated. You can feel like talking to strangers about your drinking or drug use to break the ice and to have a conversation to get along with them. With alcohol and/or drugs in common, they may seem like friends. And, all this may happen very subtly and make you feel comfortable and at ease.

## You have been reinforced for using alcohol or a drug.

Drinking alcohol and/or using drugs becomes easy to think about and notice. The importance of consuming alcohol or drugs becomes more important because of the same reinforcement. The increase in importance is a change in your values. When your values change, you come up with reasons why it is important to you. Those reasons become a way to think about using alcohol and/or drugs again. Reasons to use again help you plan to put alcohol or drugs in your body to get the good feeling of being loaded. Those same reasons will help you stand up to anyone who gets between you and using alcohol and drugs again. Reasons become a way to keep your alcohol and/or drug use hidden from those who might want to stop you.

Once you feel like using alcohol and/or a drug, it is easy to keep doing it. You have the arm and hand movements that feel right when you are consuming alcohol or drugs. You have other people who join you in the activity and socially reinforce your alcohol and/or drug use. And, of course, alcohol or drug use reinforce are reinforced with a direct brain chemistry reward every time you put it in your body. It goes right to your brain.

The punishment for using does not come close enough to the act of consuming to be a deterrent. You usually feel the problems associated with alcohol or drug use when you stop or cannot do it. Coming down is the hardest thing. But, it is the result of not using. You feel punishment for not using.

If you were arrested because of your drinking or/drug use, that was someone else who caught you. The punishment was not for drinking or drugging but for getting caught. You may think of ways not to drink and drive. You may think of better ways to buy or conceal your drug use without getting caught.

No one keeps using a substance, either alcohol or a drug, they do not like. Once you like it, you use it again. That is why they call it a brain disease of the reward center. The disease concept is that it hijacks your reward center. There is even genetic evidence to show a difference in drug liking of those who keep drinking and/or drugging after bad things happen to them as a result. The more you like it, the more reinforcing it will be to your drinking and drug use. The more you like it, the more valuable it becomes to you. The more valuable it becomes, the more reasons you have to do it again. But that also explains why you voluntarily do it.

## There is a Way Out

None of the above facts makes your hands and arms move when you do not want them to move. You can listen and observe the brain aftereffects of your alcohol and/or drug use and stop yourself from doing it again. The process also works in reverse. If you do not drink alcohol or use a drug, it will become less important to you. You can recognize your reasons to use and stop buying into them without making them go away. Alcohol and/or drugs may have conditioned you through reinforcement. You have control over that reinforcement.

Diseases do not work through reinforcement. There is nothing reinforcing about diabetes, high blood pressure, or hepatitis. You cannot quit those diseases. Alcohol and/or drug use can be quit. All recovery is about not using alcohol or drugs again. Quitting forever puts reconditioning in your hands. How do you permanently stop yourself from using alcohol and/or a drug again?

How people act when they feel like using alcohol or drugs varies depending on what is their intended outcome. It is a well-known fact that some people gain full control and never use again after being detoxed. Others haven't figured it out yet. They haven't made up their minds about whether they will use again. They will likely go and drink or use drugs again. But, they will do so because drinking and drugging was their intent. Once they make up their minds to stop, they never use again.

Someone who is under the influence of alcohol and drugs is impaired in their thinking and behavior. But, how they became under the influence was a voluntary activity. That is an important distinction that the alcohol and drug industry has lost track of. The effect on the brain from the use of alcohol and drugs is always caused by voluntary behavior when consuming after detox. If someone has not drank or used drugs and their body is in an alcohol- and drug-free state, then using is voluntary. Choosing to drink or drug again, and the act of getting the substance into one's body, are caused by voluntary actions.

The solution is found in voluntary behavior. When one no longer uses his or her hands to put alcohol and drugs into the body, the brain and body returns to its original state, unless permanent damage has been done, but that permanent damage is not of the nature that prevents the person from abstaining. As a matter of fact, there is no line to be crossed where we can ever know that a person who is using has transitioned from voluntary to involuntary use. There is nothing to be found psychologically or physically to determine involuntary behavior has taken place. So, how can anyone with sound reasoning say someone's drug or alcohol use took place involuntarily? Telling people they use involuntarily because of their addiction gives them the excuse to use the word relapse.

# The Brain-Recovery Model: Who Controls Your Hands?

How do you know that if you want to keep yourself from using again, you can carry it out for the remainder of your life? How can quitting forever be possible?

This is basically how your brain and body work together. You just learned what you did to your brain and how you can let it return to its natural state. This is why you know you can keep your hands from picking up alcohol or drugs, even after changing your brain chemistry and conditioning yourself.

There are three parts of the brain I want you to remember: the forebrain with the cortex, the midbrain with the midbrain with the VTA (Ventral Tegmentum, and the hindbrain the most primitive part of the brain controlling heart beat and breathing. I am going to teach you the structure and function of the brain. Alcohol and drugs affect your body and brain. You need to understand the way your body and brain work together, so you can get out of this. You can look this up in any anatomy of biology book. It will be more complex, so I am teaching an easier way to understand it. Your brain has many parts, and they all work together.

**Structure.** Your midbrain and hindbrain are under the cortex and extend down to the end of your brain stem. The hindbrain is the most primitive part of your brain. It includes the limbic system, which controls emotional behavior.

The cortex is the modern part of your brain. Your cortex is above and all around the midbrain. The brain stem runs up and down your spinal column, with nerves and neurons that run to your arms and legs. The neurons from your cortex to your arms are about three feet long. They are directly connected to your arms and legs from your sensory motor cortex. If you cut those nerves, you would lose movement, because that part of your brain would no longer be directly connected to your arms.

The midbrain contains an endogenous reward system using the structures of the VTA and the nucleus accumbens which send neurons to the prefrontal cortex. Endogenous means within or inside the midbrain. The reward system words subset of its own as a structure.

**Function.** The primitive midbrain and hind brain are old lower brain structures that evolved very early in time. Lizards and animals have large mid and hindbrain areas compared to their cortex. The hindbrain controls involuntary functions and allows for survival. Involuntary functions include heartbeat, respiration or breathing, appetite, and pupil dilation. You emotions are created in this area. It is like a control panel for an automatic pilot. It is just there doing its job. It has no sense of time and no self concept. Self concept is where you can say to yourself, "I am I and you are you and not me." Self concept is the words you use to label yourself and the story you use to understand yourself. The lower brain function is just to keep your body alive and to survive.

Part of its survival job is to get you to consume things you need to stay alive, like breathing air, drinking water, and eating food. Remember, appetites are located in your midbrain endogenous pleasure pathway. The reward pathway helps you orient yourself and pay attention to things you need to stay alive. It can only say yes to consume things you need to stay alive. It cannot say no. Your pleasure center is located in your reward pathway of the midbrain area. The pleasure center and reward pathway makes things seem satisfying. It says, "I want more of that." That is why food and water can be so satisfying and give you pleasure. That is the basic function of the lower brain.

The modern cortex is all around the mid and hindbrain. It completely surrounds it on the top and sides. Cortex is the modern brain. The cortex is the thinking part of the brain. It is the self concept in you. The cortex is where your identity lies because of the self concept. Your identity is how you think of yourself. The cortex is also an inhibitor. It can say yes or no. It gives you the ability to say yes or no because the cortex is voluntary (volitional). It controls voluntary functions. The muscles in your arms and legs are voluntary muscles. You move your limbs by extending and contracting voluntary muscles when they receive signals sent via nerves from the sensory motor part of the cortex. Remember, there is a special part of your cortex that controls movement. That part is called the sensory motor cortex. You have to learn to maneuver your hand on the end of your arm through time and space in order to pick something up. You use vision and the feeling sensation to judge how hard it is to grasp something and to judge how much force to use to pick it up. Without learning to use that complex ability, and without a lot of self-control, you could not pick up anything. Motor movement is planned in the cortex. You choose what movement you should make next. There is an orderly representation of the body on the motor cortex. A lot more area of the motor cortex is devoted to your hands and fingers because they are involved in complex movement.

## Bring It Back to Drinking Alcohol and Using Drugs

Let us bring it back to addiction. When you use substances like alcohol and drugs, you stimulate the pleasure pathways of the midbrain, especially the pleasure part of it in the reward pathway. You feel a pleasure reward. Once you use that substance, you know that it will make you feel pleasure. You know it will give you that good, buzz feeling. There is a certain loaded feeling that you come to love. That is why you do it again, because it feels so good. But, that is the only reason you do it again. You not only like that feeling, you come to love it. Drinking and/or drugging become very important to you. It becomes important enough to compete with activities and people your love.

People can use a substance that stimulates that pleasure center and never become addicted. Two things have to happen to become addicted: you have to use the substance and like the way it makes you feel, and you have to use it again and again to that level of intoxication you grow to love. With powerful drugs like heroin and amphetamines, you don't have to use much of it to get to that intoxication level that feels really good.

You habituate to it really quickly, so you start to get a physical dependency. That is the only reason you use the stuff again and again. A nerve goes from the VTA of your midbrain into the prefrontal cortex to send signals saying it wants alcohol or drugs again. That is why you notice when alcohol and drugs are present and why think about alcohol and drugs without trying.

# Brain Recovery Model

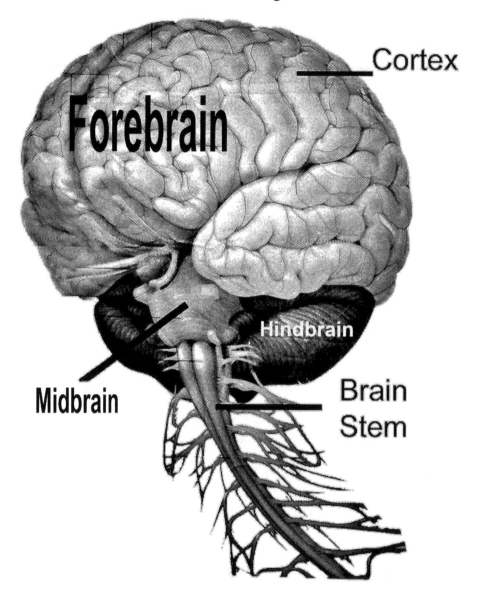

Remember three different parts of the brain: forebrain with the cortex, midbrain with the reward pathway and hindbrain with the survival system. The primitive lower brain areas evolved early and are the control panel for involuntary movement and functions. It is the automatic control panel for your pleasure pathway. It can only say, "Yes, consume things you need to stay alive, like oxygen, food, and water." It has no sense of time and no self concept. Emotion and pleasure centers are located here. When you drink alcohol and/or use drugs, you stimulate the pleasure center and form a hunger for the substance. You fall in love with the buzz or the high the substance stimulates, and you want to return to the feeling of pleasure by seeking out alcohol and drugs. To become addicted, you have to return repeatedly to that preferred level of high. You come to look forward to getting loaded and anticipate pleasure by thinking about it.

People can use a substance that stimulates that pleasure center and never become addicted. Two things have to happen to become addicted: you have to use the substance and like the way it makes you feel, and you have to use it again and again to that level of intoxication you grow to love. With powerful drugs like heroin and amphetamines, you don't have to use much of it to get to that intoxication level that feels really good. You habituate to it really quickly, so you start to get a physical dependency. That is the only reason you use the stuff again and again. A nerve goes from the VTA of your midbrain into the prefrontal cortex to send signals saying it wants alcohol or drugs again. That is why you notice when alcohol and drugs are present and why think about alcohol and drugs without trying.

Some substance abuse counselors say you drink alcohol or used drugs because of your problems and genetics, but that is not the reason you keep using. Did anyone test you genetically to see if you had the gene for addiction? If they did not test you genetically, it was like malpractice for anyone with a license to diagnose you as an addict because of your genetic heritage.

Problems that you have do not make you use. You do not run from problems, you run to intoxication. You only run to the intoxication that you have tried and fallen in love with. Antidepressants will solve your problem of feeling depressed. But that won't stop you from drinking and using drugs, because your problems are not why you are using. You use alcohol and/or drugs to stimulate the reward pathway pleasure center in your midbrain and return to that wonderful feeling of intoxication that you have grown to love. Basically, that is where addiction comes from; it is that and nothing but that. I am not saying that you do not have problems, and I don't know about your genetic makeup, but they do not make you use alcohol and drugs when you do not want to use alcohol and drugs.

## Why You Can Keep Yourself from Drinking and Drugs

Let's get away from addiction and talk about recovery by quitting forever. This is about never using again. Remember the original question? How do you know that if you want to keep yourself from using again you can carry it out for the remainder of your life? They say there is no guarantee. I can show you why there is a guarantee.

When you trace the nerves from the midbrain VTA, they go to the prefrontal cortex. The nerves do not go from the rewarding pleasure pathways directly to the sensory motor cortex. There is no direct connection. The connection is by association only. I say it again so please remember, the nerves from the lower brain only go to the prefrontal cortex and they don't go to the sensory motor cortex. There are no nerves that connect the midbrain, the part that wants the substance, with the part of the brain that controls your hands. So, how can that desire, that part of your brain that wants the substance, make you pick it up? It cannot! It is biologically impossible.

If you make a decision to never pick up alcohol and drugs again, you would not pick it up unless you changed your mind. If you made up your mind and stuck to it, could that feeling to use ever make you pick it up? No! Even if we put your favorite drink or drug within reach in front of you; and seeing it stimulates your rewarding pleasure pathway system so you really want alcohol or a drug, and you feel shaky and maybe sweat, and your tongue hangs out for it. Can that make you pick it up? No! That experience cannot directly make you pick it up. Why not?

Your body and brain do not work that way. It is biologically impossible for your hungry pleasure pathway in the midbrain to force you to pick up alcohol or drugs when you refuse to move your hands, because there is no direct connection to make you do it against your decision and values to abstain.

You can resolve your ambivalence, make up your mind with a decision, and carry out your decision in the face of your lower brain calling out for you to use alcohol or drugs. Once you know and accept what has happened, you don't have to struggle. You know what is going on. Feeling your pleasure pathway calling can have a different meaning than you feel like drinking or using drugs. The feeling can have no meaning instead of feeling like drinking or using drugs; it can just awareness you are feeling a sensation.

So, when they tell you drinking and drug use happens outside your control, you can see that biological loss of control before you initially drink or use drugs makes no-sense. With that in place, can you give yourself a virtual guarantee that you will never use again? Yes you can, and without a doubt. As long as you don't change your mind about not using, you will never pick it up. Changing your mind does not mean you will never have feelings and thoughts again about drinking alcohol or using a drug. Those are internal experiences largely beyond your control from occurring. What not changing your mind means you will follow your values of quitting forever never using by controlling your external experience of moving your arms and hands to pick the stuff and put them in your body. The feeling to use will become less and less as the result of not using. Some emotional memories may remain, but you do not have to fight, run from, or control those feelings. Research has shown brain cells can recover from damage caused by alcohol and drugs after a period of time. You will never become high or intoxicated again if you never pick up and drink or use again.

You will be recovered because of quitting forever. You can get more detox, and your brain may take some time to return to its natural state, but you will not be more recovered. Recovery happens the moment quitting forever takes place and you never use again. Recovery has to start at some point in time to happen. You know you have not recovered if you are not sure about using drugs or drinking again. You have recovered if you never again drink alcohol or use drugs. You know you are done quitting forever because of your experience when you feel like using. You feel pleased you are not drinking and drugging and are confident you will remain because of quitting forever.

You may have problems in your life that remain to be solved. You may have interpersonal problems and find it difficult to get along with other people. You may have difficulty asserting yourself. Emotional problems may go away, or you may continue to have difficulty with emotion regulation. Health problems may require medical attention. Practical problems like finding a job, or a better job, remain. Let those things be separate from your recovery. Solve those problems, so your life will be better because they are solved. You never drink or use drugs no matter what problems you have or how difficult they are to solve.

# Brain Recovery Model

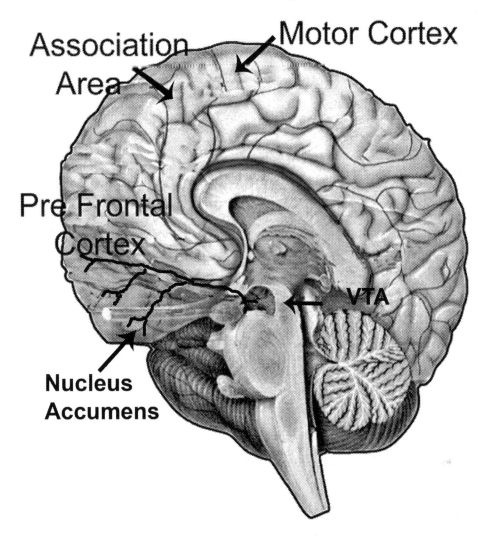

The reason you can recover from alcohol and drugs is because there is no direct nerve connection between the prefrontal cortex and the motor cortex. The pleasure pathway of the midbrain can hijack the cortex when you become addicted. The VTA of the midbrain sends out signals via nerves to the prefrontal cortex responsible for planning, choosing, and decision making. The cortex can say yes or no and is known as the inhibitor. There is a special part of the cortex, the sensory motor cortex that controls voluntary movement. You have to plan to move your hands and feet for them to move. You have to make your limbs move in order for them to move. You do not pick up things unless you have the intent to pick them up. You are aware of that intent and then carry out that intent with your sensory motor cortex. Once you learn what is going on, you can experience the midbrain stimulating the prefrontal cortex and telling you to pick up alcohol or drugs, but you will still not pick them up because you override lower brain with a decision. Your lower brain can no longer hijack your cortex unless you change your decision. You don't change decisions involuntarily but only after thinking about it. Your lower brain can never directly make you pick up alcohol or drugs.

# Solve problems so your life will be better.
# Do not solve problems to keep yourself from drinking or drugging

What we want to talk about is how to not change your mind. Now that you know you are not going to lose control of your arms and hands, will that stop your midbrain from calling out for the intoxicating substance you used to feed it? Will the midbrain still desire it? Of course it will. It will signal your prefrontal cortex send you memories of fun you had while loaded. Your prefrontal cortex will talk to you about using. It will remind you it is time to use. It will show you pictures inside your head about the substance. It will direct your attention to the sight and smell of it. It will focus in on other people drinking and drugging and tell you how much fun they are having. If you try to reason with your brain, it will deliberate with you and strike a reasonable bargain to get you to drink or use impulsively. You can get away with it this time. Nothing bad will happen. You won't get caught. No one will know. Do not try to stop those thoughts from happening, or you will be struggling with them. It is when you observe those thoughts happening but give them no value that you are freed. Let those thoughts and feelings flow through your mind like a leaf falling off a tree, drifting down to a stream that carries them away. Trying not to think about it will make you think about it. You will not go back on your decision after quitting forever by willingly controlling what is external, your hands. You do not have to battle with your internal feelings anymore. You know what you are going to do and you do not control the stream of chattering thoughts going through your head.

# The Test

Some people thinking about quitting forever talk about a time in the future when they will be tested. They wonder if they will pass the test. One of the tests is, "What will I do when they [legal system, parents, significant other, promise to friend or doctor, whoever is stopping you] are no longer requiring me to not drink or use drugs?" The other type of test is the special event test. "How do I know I will not drink [use drugs] on New Year's [birthday, holiday, or death of a loved one] until I am in that situation." In both instances, the person wonders how one can know what he or she will do until confronted by such an event. There is a test, but you do not have to take it.

What is meant by a test? A test is a condition leading to proof. When you take a test, you are asked to demonstrate a skill to be evaluated. When you produce the skill, you demonstrate proof you can do it and pass the test. You are usually given a chance to study or practice before you take a test. You are told to learn the material and practice a skill. For example, if you are going to take a driver's test, you learn the rules of the road and what the road signs mean. You practice steering and breaking and move from driving in a parking lot to driving in traffic. Then, you are given a written test to show you have learned the material before you are given a driver's test to show you have the behavioral skills. You do not know what will be on the written test, and you do not know what they will have you do on the driver's test. Since you do not know what you will be asked or required to do, then you do not know what you will answer or what you will do when tested.

The nature of a test is you do not know if you will pass until you take the test. You can know you have studied and practiced a skill or a set of skills. But, you do not know the result of the test until tested. Will the questions be worded in a way hard to understand? Will there be trick maneuvers requiring movements you are unfamiliar with? Test taking usually is a time of anticipation and anxiety about the results of the test. Some people worry about tests so much they have what is called test anxiety. Test anxiety is where someone feels excessive worry when faced with the idea of having to take a test. A person who has test anxiety usually has failed a test before and felt really bad afterward. They are now afraid about the prospect of being tested again, because they do not want to feel bad again.

**Here is the test.** Not drinking or using drugs is a test if you are not using one day at a time or are trying to prevent relapse. One day at a time means you have said you will not drink or not use drugs today, but you are not sure about after today. Every day is another test to see if you have the strength or determination to make up your mind not to drink or drug for today, but tomorrow, you will be tested again. What will you do and how do you know what you will do until that day comes? You truly do not know what you will do. Your mind is not made up about what you will do. How do you know how you will feel and what will be going on in your life? Not drinking or drugging will be dependent on what is going on and if you can choose to not drink or drug for that day. And, you better be able to get to your group or call your sponsor and get someone to help you before you drink or drug. You will be tested to see if you can come up with enough reasons not to drink or use drugs today. You will be tested, and you wonder if you will pass. You may have test anxiety.

With relapse prevention, you can never know if you are going to relapse and if you can prevent it from happening. You have to remember your list of reasons not to drink or drug when you feel like doing it. You have to be able to recognize your triggers and avoid or cope with them. You have to be able to recognize apparently irrelevant situations and decisions so you don't drink or drug. You better be able to change the thoughts in your mind and the feeling to drink or drug when you feel like doing it. You will have to do all that when you feel like drinking or doing drugs. You will be tested every time you feel like drinking or using. The test can make you feel anxious.

Would you like to know how to get out of the test? Is not drinking (or using a drug) after quitting forever still a test? After quitting forever, you do not use your hands to pick up alcohol or drugs to put them into your body. When faced with alcohol or drugs, there is no special hand movement to be remembered. You know the question on the test: will you drink alcohol or use a drug? You know the correct answer: never. The question will never change, and the answer is always the same. You control your hands, and they will not move to pick up alcohol or a drug unless you make them move. You have that behavioral ability. What other test is there where you know the question, the answer is one word, and the behavior is not moving your hands to pick up alcohol or drugs? You may not have completed quitting forever if you feel anxious about what you are going to do. You do not feel anxious about whether you are going to drink or drug after quitting forever although you may feel anxiety about other things. Plenty of people feel anxious about a lot of things and still control their hands after quitting forever.

You do not have to change anything after quitting forever. There is no test of your ability to change anything. You knew you were going to feel like drinking or drugging again at some time. You knew you may feel anxious about the thought or feeling of drinking or drugging. That is happening to you right now. You accept the thoughts and feelings and let them pass without fighting them, because they have no value to you. They are just thoughts and feelings, not things that guide your action. You do not have to avoid them or make them go away. You have felt them before; you are feeling them again. You know you are not going to drink or use drugs. Picking up alcohol or drugs and using them would be making a change. There is nothing to change after quitting forever. You knew you were not going to pick up or use alcohol and/or drugs before you felt this way. You know the feeling will pass. Where is the test? There is nothing to prove.

You may feel like you are going to be tested if you have doubt about quitting forever. If someplace inside there is knowledge that you may not be using because someone will punish you, then you may wonder what you would do if you would not get punished. The thoughts of wonder may sound something like this. "What will I do when there is no impending punishment if I drink alcohol or use drugs? I have not faced that question in myself. It feels uncomfortable to face that and decide before it happens. I can't make up my mind what I will do. How do I know what I will do until faced with the situation when I will not be punished when I feel like drinking or drugging and have the opportunity to do it?" That surely is a test. It is a big test with pass-fail results. You may feel anxious because you are waiting to see what you will do to prove to yourself you will not drink or drug. Not drinking or using drugs at that time may not be enough to prove anything to you. It will only be enough proof if, when you do not drink or drug, it is because of quitting forever. But, it is a test.

Not facing your doubt about quitting forever is risky. If you cannot face your indecision about what you will do now, how will you be better able to face those feelings when you are under pressure to make up your mind at that time? You may want to avoid your indecision right now because it is uncomfortable and difficult to think about, but you cannot avoid forever. You will have to choose what to do under the pressure of your internal feeling of drinking or drugging and external cues triggering you to drink or drug. And, there will be external time pressure, because if you do not choose to drink or drug, you will be left out of what other people are doing if you take too long to decide you want to drink or use drugs. What are you going to do? You may not know until you are in the situation. But, you will be tested by the situation.

There are two ways to get out of the test. One way is decide you will drink or use drugs when you are presented with them and feel like doing it. There will be no test of whether you can keep yourself from doing it because you have decided to use when the situation presents itself. There will be a different kind of test. This will test your ability to pick a situation where you will not get in trouble for your drinking or drugging. Can you keep from drinking or drugging too much or for too long a time? Will it be safe to do it this time or not? Will you keep yourself from driving, spending too much money, or doing something that is beneath your values or moral code once you used? It may seem safe, but it is a risk; you do not know what will happen. You will be tested. And you will keep being tested, because you will be drinking and drugging again after this time. You will feel anxious about watching yourself reach for alcohol or drugs, but it will go away once you are loaded again. It may not stay away even if you are loaded, because you may fear getting caught if they drive or have to take a drug test.

The other way is to decide you will never drink or use drugs when you feel like doing it. Unconditional quitting forever ends tests without risk of ever being drunk or high again. This is not about you and other people who will punish you. Avoiding punishment is conditional quitting, and it is not forever but based on avoiding bad things happening, things like bad health, wasted money, and any other thing you can imagine. The possibility exists that you could be convinced you will not get in trouble.

Quitting forever based on conditions is indecision and doubt about what you will do. If quitting forever only means avoiding bad consequences, you have not made up your mind about quitting forever, no matter what the consequences. Remember, avoiding consequences may be a reason for quitting forever. If after quitting forever, you are using any reasons

other than quitting forever, it is not unconditional. Unconditional means you never drink or use drugs, even if only good things will happen. Using good and bad reasons to drink or drug or not to drink or drug keeps you reasoning and thinking about drinking or using drugs. If you have to use reasons for not drinking or using drugs other than quitting forever, you will be tested. If you are using reasons, it is similar to one day at a time or relapse prevention. Can you come up with the reasons, or do you need someone to help you? You will be tested. You can get out of the test by ending reasons.

Quitting forever ends reasoning or deliberating about why you will not drink or use drugs. Quitting forever is the reason. You do not feel like you will be tested, because you know what you will always do. Not drinking or using drugs works well in all situations and in all environments. There is nothing to learn to control, because there are no special hand movements. You have had a lifetime of experience using your hands and arms, and you know you never pick up anything you do not intend to pick up. Your intention and values are clear because of quitting forever. You never pick up alcohol or drugs, even when those old familiar thoughts or feelings come back. You already accepted them and know they do not control your hands. You do not have to make them go away, because they have no value to you. It does not seem like a test; this is the way you do it from now on. You are done after quitting forever. You will never be tested again about whether you are going to drink or use drugs. There is no test to pass.

## Thoughts to Use Will Continue After Quitting Forever

Get in touch with them right now. Right now is this moment in time. Feel your eyes blink, and let them close when you are comfortable. Feel the seat underneath you. Notice the position of your hands. Is there a noticeable odor in the room? Focus on your breathing. Follow it in and out without changing your breathing patterns. Catch your breath and breathe easily. Notice the thoughts in your head. Notice any sensations going though your body. That is what is going on in the moment of right now.

Value is when something is important or means something to you. When you notice thoughts and sensations, you can buy into them and make them important to you. You can analyze their meaning. You can argue with them and dispute them. All that will keep you engaged with the chatter in your mind. All that has a place, but you pick the time and place. It is natural to be aware of words and sensations when they arise. That is part of being human. We often take the ongoing stream of thoughts and sensations too literally when it is better observed as mind chatter and not meaningful to following our values.

Return to the thoughts and feelings you are aware of right now. Let them be there without giving them any meaning. They are in your head and awareness, but you can let them pass without buying into them. Observe them for what they are: thoughts and sensations. They are not commands to be defied or gotten rid of. That is fighting your inner experience. Do not retreat from your inner experience or sustain it. Make room for it to be there just as it is a thought and a feeling. They are thoughts and feelings that do not control your hands. Your values control your hands. You know what you are going to do without being influenced by the chatter in your mind. Fighting the chatter will make it come back more often and stronger. Alcohol and drug treatment teaches you how to fight you inner experience. The twelve steps will have you avoid it by going to groups and talking with your sponsor. Rational Recovery will have you battle it like a beast in your mind. Cognitive behavioral therapists will teach you how to distract yourself. Relapse prevention will have you come up with reasons why you should not drink or use. SMART recovery and Rational Emotive Behavioral Therapy will have you dispute your thoughts. Quitting forever means you know how to move beyond all of that. You will stop battling automatic thoughts to use and not try to make them go away. You accept them as there because you used drugs or drank alcohol. They have no current meaning to you. Just chatter. Let them be. Who controls your hands?

## Learn a Set of Skills Where You Will Be Successful All the Time

Do you have reoccurring slips and relapses back to alcohol and drug use? Chronic use may be more a function of interacting with recovery movement providers than the aftereffects of being addicted to alcohol or drugs. Get detoxed to get the alcohol or drugs out of your body. Then ask yourself, "What am I recovering from?" You repeatedly used the substance, so you are recovering from the act of using as well as from the effects of the substance. One follows the other. Ask yourself, "Do I want to make sure this will never happen again?"

What has been your recovery experience to date? Were you overwhelmed and left struggling and living with slips and relapses? Did you feel coerced to attend twelve-step groups? Did you feel deceived when you were told that AA or NA groups were not religious but only spiritual? Have you returned to your previous level of alcohol or drug use? What were the most helpful and the least helpful parts of your experience with the recovery industry? People are often advised to take what they want and to leave the rest. Often some of the things they were taught in their recovery experience that they took and seemed helpful were actually harmful.

The parts you left because they seem harmful probably were. Counting time clean and sober, one day at a time, and the disease model of addiction are harmful. The idea that recovery has something to do with attending groups, that you need to be humbled, and that you must have a sponsor are harmful. The phrase "never say never" is not only harmful, it is self-contradictory. The idea that your own best thinking got you here is not only harmful but also insulting. You may have been told to that to remain abstinent, you must lead your life like a second-class citizen, staying away from places where alcohol or drugs might be available.

Think about never using alcohol and drugs again, and listen to what pops into your head. If you are quitting forever, then you better start thinking about the idea. What ideas do you have about not quitting? Say to yourself, "I will never use alcohol or drugs again." What do you feel? Does it sound like a lie to you? There lies the problem. You may not be absolutely sure you never want to drink or drug again. Or, you may doubt your ability to carry out never using. When you think about never using again, do you also think about using again? So, go ahead. Right now, while you are reading about quitting forever, make a conscious plan to use alcohol or drugs again. Do you really want to carry that out, or do you think about not using alcohol or drugs? Do you feel uneasy about the idea of planning to use? If you listen, you will hear yourself thinking both ways, going back and forth between two sets of ideas. You likely are ambivalent about what you will do. If you are still choosing what to do, perhaps your mind is not made up about what you are going to do when it comes to alcohol or drugs. The basic fact is that you have to make up your mind. No one can do it for you. It has to be one way or the other. Either you will use again or you will abstain. But, right now, you may not be sure what you will do. Twelve steppers and counselors may have even yelled at you, saying you can never predict what you will do in the future when it comes to alcohol or drugs. Remember, when people have an organized plan, it can be difficult to change that plan.

# What is the difference between a choice and a decision?

A choice is when you are presented with two options and you have to pick one or the other to do. A decision is something that is made ahead of time and you are waiting to do. When you have a choice, it is one or the other. You have to make that choice by picking. A decision is already made. You don't have to make a choice and pick once you have made a decision. The choice is already made in a decision.

A choice is something you are going to have to do at some point in time. But, a decision no longer depends on time. A choice comes when you are faced with a choice point. At some point in time, you have to do one thing or you will be doing the other. You can't do both when it comes to drinking and drugging and not drinking and drugging. One eliminates the other. You will be faced with a choice, and you will have to pick which one to do. That is what makes it a choice. You are either going to do one or the other and that will be at a point in time that one eliminated the other choice. You can't do both.

Don't be confused by the terminology. When you are making a choice, you are making a short term decision for this time. At the choice point, you deliberate back and forth and decide which one to pick as your choice. But, when you make a choice, it means you haven't made a decision ahead of time. You have not made your decision if you are choosing. It is the choosing that results in deciding which one to pick. But, that is not the type of decision I was originally referring to. In the decision I originally referred to, you have already made your mind up about not drinking or drugging before the choice point. It was a previously made decision, and there is no anticipation about choice once a decision is made. In a decision, there is no need for anticipation at the choice point. The anticipation was done long ago, and the decision is just carried out as a behavior you do at the choice point.

What does that mean to you when it comes to drinking or using drugs? If you have not made the decision you are never going to drink again and someone put a drink in front of you, you had to make a choice of whether to pick it up. You struggle choosing. If you had already made the decision not to drink, then you wouldn't have to pick and choose about what you were going to do. No struggling. See the difference in what I mean between a choice and a decision?

Let me diagram it out to help clarify it. First, let me diagram a choice. There is a timeline with a choice point. At some point on the timeline, you come to a fork where there is more than one way to go. You will have to pick one or the other. There has to be at least A or B. You are going to have to deliberate and decide which one to pick in order to make your choice. During the anticipation time on the timeline, you don't know which one you will pick. Your anticipation is that you will have to pick but not which one you will pick. You are ambivalent. Ambivalent means you are attracted and repelled by both options. To make a choice, your mind can't be made up until you reach the choice point. You don't really know what you are going to do. Ambivalence may have you going back and forth in anticipation of which choice you will make. No predetermined decision is yet made. You are waiting for the choice point to choose. You are waiting through time to figure out what you will do. You are waiting in anticipation of the choice point. The two choices are mutually exclusive in that if you drink or use drugs now then you have not quit and the longer you wait you will not be drinking or drugging. You cannot both drink and drug and not drink and drug at the same time. You have to do the other one.

For example, if it is drinking or using drugs, at some point in time you have put the substance into your body. You just used. At some point, it is too late to drink; you will be at home in bed asleep. But, when you wake up, you will have to choose all over again, and it may be a different choice next time. You will never know what you are going to choose in the future as long as you keep choosing. You can't drink and abstain. If you drink even a sip, you are drinking. It is not the amount. Drinking and/or drug use is something that is mutually exclusive. You either do it or not do it. It is black or white, with no shades of gray. It is one or the other. There is no gradient. You are not quibbling over the amount. Any amount was a choice to do it. This is not a bargain of how much. That is too complicated and gets you back to words in your head. Can you see all the elements that have been presented in a choice so far?

## Decide, and You Know What You are Doing Before Choosing.

Let me diagram a decision. A decision looks similar to a choice when you draw it. There is still a timeline. And there has to be more than one way to go. There is still an A and B option to pick. But, the decision ends the deliberation. A decision ends deciding and choosing. A decision ends the anticipation, because it is made in advance of the choice point. A decision is made indeed. The decision was A and not B. If it is a big decision or a strong decision, you decide it will always be A and never B. Now, you continue along in time. You are faced with a choice point. Do you have to figure out which one to pick? No, you do not. Why not? Because, you have already decided. You picked ahead of time. Was there anything to figure out after the decision was made? No. Is there anything to argue with yourself over or ever question after you make an important decision? No. Do you want to continue to weigh the consequences of good and bad or benefit and harm after you made your decision? No. That is ambivalence about the decision if

# Difference Between a Choice And a Decision

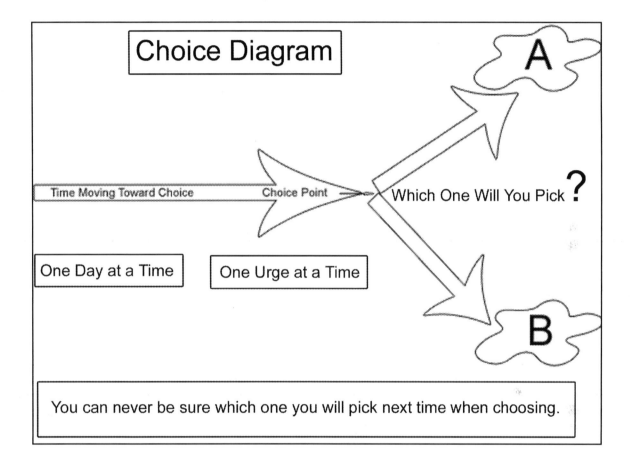

Think about what a choice is. You have been thinking about making a choice to drink or drug or wait until later. Are you going to buy into the words in your head? Some of the words are about using. You are digging a hole.

When you make a choice, you do not know which option you will select when you get to the choice point. You deliberate options to make your choice and then pick one. The deliberation is like ambivalence. Each segment in the timeline brings you closer to the choice point where you have a preference for A or you will be doing B. Your choices are a pragmatic absolute, because there are no other alternatives. You have to elect one or get the other by default.

not accepted as automatic mind chatter. Ambivalence means you bought into the thoughts that you have not decided and that you are still choosing. If you made a decision, there is no question of what you will do because you are not caught up in your mind you are caught up in carrying out a decision you made based on your values. And if that decision was for always, then you will never revisit this issue. You always know what you are going to do. We could go on in time and let you face the same choice point again and again. If you made a decision, would it make any difference? No, it is always the same, and it doesn't take a lot of thinking, brains, or willpower to carry it out. There is nothing to figure out, think about, or second-guess. You don't get caught up in your mind. You get caught up in your values and your actions.

What about with a choice? Is there anything to figure out think about or second-guess? Yes there is, and it keeps you forever figuring it out. That is what one day at a time and relapse prevention does to you. Choosing is like AA and NA. If you choose for one day, isn't there the next day when you have to choose again? What will you do that day or sometime in the future? You don't know and will never know for sure. Does it make any difference if you are thinking of the next day, next week, next month, year, or some imaginary time in the future? If you don't know what you are going to do, then you don't know. That is one of the problems with the recovery movement. It never lets you make up your mind and keeps you unresolved about a choice point you will face again and again.

People drink or use drugs again for two reasons. One is they never made up their mind that they would not do it anymore. They never decided. They never said to themselves, "I will never do it again." They said it to other people. Sure, they would say it to other people to get those other people off their back. Or, they say it quickly and impulsively, without really thinking about or contemplating quitting forever. "What does this really mean to me? Do I really mean forever, or is it that I just feel so sick and sorry about this that I wish it would go away right now? OK, I will never drink or use drugs again." Or, was it really thought out? "Wait a minute. What am I really saying to myself, and who am I promising? How important is this decision to me? I am not promising anyone else, just myself. This is a long time. It really does mean forever. Do I really want to never use alcohol and drugs again?" You don't have to ask yourself that question again and again until you know the answer. You have to make up your mind what you will do to resolve your ambivalence. Until then, your reason may be following not directing.

To repeat, one reason someone drinks or drugs again is because they never really quit to themselves to begin with. And if they did quit to themselves, then the second reason they drink or use again is they later changed their mind. They didn't really make it that serious, where the decision was unchangeable. They went back to weighing consequences in the form of deliberation. They got caught up in their mind and considered drinking alcohol or using drugs and bought into the idea to carry out the behavior. They started thinking of it as a choice and returned to choosing. Choosing left them ambivalent and not knowing what they would do, drink alcohol and/or use drugs or abstain. They were open to changing their mind. They began to question their decision and left it open to pick a new answer. They began to wonder what they would do. They got caught up in the words and in their mind that remembers drinking alcohol and using drugs.

# Difference Between a Choice and a Decision

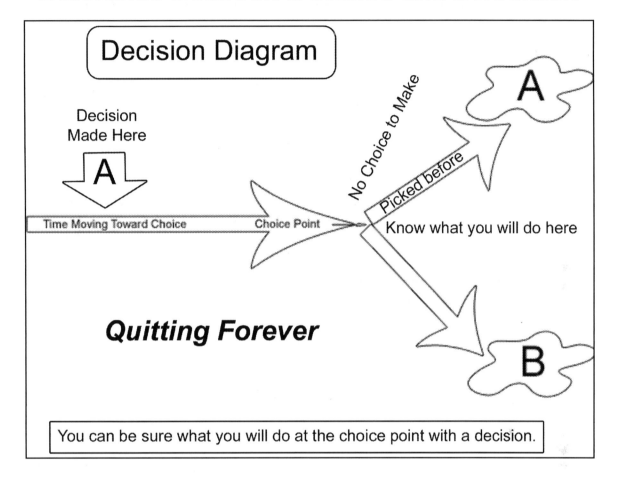

When you make a decision, you know which option you will select when you reach the choice point. You considered both options and your conclusion is never B. With the conclusion, there is nothing more to deliberate, and you are not ambivalent. Your preference is predetermined. There is nothing to choose at the choice point. Your mind is made up because of the decision. You are resolved as to what you will do before you ever reach the choice point. Knowing what you will do at the choice point after a decision is made is a skill you can learn, carry out, and get good at performing. You can become self-confident in your ability to abstain from alcohol and drugs because of a decision.

People start drinking or using drugs again because they started thinking about using again in a way that was deliberating. They considered re-deciding. They were uncomfortable about having thoughts and feelings to drink and/or use drugs without using. Remember, the midbrain is not capable of moving your hands. It can only send signals to the prefrontal cortex. Deliberating is a form of ambivalence based on a signal from VTA of the midbrain. Stop trying to control your thoughts and discomfort and only control your hands. Your decision will remain the way you made it by controlling your hands.

---

## A decision ends anticipation, because it is made in advance of the choice point.

---

Once you have thought about whether you want to quit forever, if the answer is yes, ask yourself when you will carry out what is necessary. "It needs to be done, now, when will I do it? When will I say to myself, right now and hereafter from now on, I never drink alcohol or use drugs again? Any day and time will do. The time to stop will always be the present time.

Quitting forever means that you will do three things: (1) you will never pick up alcohol or drugs and put them into your body again; (2) you will stop deliberating about whether you are ever going to use alcohol or drugs again by accepting your thoughts and feeling to drink and not drink as they occurs and just rely on the fact that you have quit; (3) you will have the experience of wanting to drink and/or drug, you observer yourself having that experience accepting it without giving it meaning, and you will use your skill of controlling your hands. You made the decision carrying it out is all that matters after quitting forever.

Why do you have to keep making up your mind if your mind is made up? You stop yourself from arguing about not using because you know it was done. There are no longer two sides to the issue. There is only one side, never. You decided never drink alcohol or use drugs no matter how you feel or what the drinking or drugging opportunity or occasion.

---

## Don't get caught up in choosing

---

# Quitting Forever: There are four areas of readiness to change:

Take a sheet of paper and write the answers to the following questions.
Read your answers again on another day.

**Need**: Do you see a reason to change your drinking and/or drug use?

What ways are you still satisfied with your alcohol and/or drug use?

What ways have you become dissatisfied with your alcohol and/or drug use?

Can you have what you are satisfied with without what you are dissatisfied with?

What is your perspective about getting drunk and stoned like you have been doing? Before you say where you want to be, think about where you are in your life because of drinking and drugs and how you feel about where you are in your life.

**Commitment to change:** What do you think will happen if you never drink or use drugs again?

Will it make your life better? Are you prepared to abstain if your life does not get better?

Do you have the desire to quit alcohol and drugs forever? Do you think that you have the ability to carry it out, or are you filled with doubts?

What are your expectations when it comes to living without alcohol and drugs?

What hope do you have for the future?

Who are the people in your life that you see supporting you in your abstinence?

How much support do you think you need?

**Awareness of self:** Are you aware of the words in your mind to use alcohol and/or drugs, or do you see it as just all you?

What are your values when it comes to further use of alcohol and/or drugs and lifelong abstinence?

Can you recognize that you have both thoughts to use and thoughts to abstain?

What ways do you value self-responsibility and self-reliance?

Can you hear yourself going back and forth between the idea of drinking and/or using and abstaining?

Can you willingly shift back and forth between the two sets of ideas? Can you hold the idea of never drinking or using drugs in your mind while you feel the desire for alcohol and drugs?

Can you recognize thoughts, feelings, and images to use drugs and alcohol as something that is part of you and accept it while you abstain? Are you someone who can make up your mind and keep it that way because of your values?

Can you understand that making up your mind is a skill that can be learned if you have the desire and commitment of quitting forever?

**Awareness of your environment:** Do you know that alcohol and drugs will not go away because of quitting forever?

Are you ready to recognize and deal with alcohol and drugs being in your community while you abstain?

Do you understand that you cannot hide from alcohol and drugs?

Can you really be sure that no one will ever offer you alcohol and drugs again as long as you live?

Are you ready to abstain when really good alcohol and drugs are offered cheaply or for free?

Are there any special days of the year when using alcohol or drugs will be the exception to your abstinence?

## Summary and Review

You were given explicit instructions on quitting forever at the beginning of this book. I divulged how I derived the book *The Natural Process of Quitting Forever: Explicit Instruction*, showing I did not just make it up. The information was there, available for anyone to put together if they could see quitting forever as possible. One-day-at-a-time advice was considered in comparison to quitting forever. Informed consent gave you an opportunity to think about some of the side effects of quitting forever. I insist I am not criticizing institutions in total. I am only criticizing information that runs counter to or that discourages someone from quitting forever.

I showed you quitting forever is a natural thing to do as opposed to taking a supernatural, tentative, unsure course of action. Myths in alcohol and drug recovery were revealed. The principles and values of quitting forever were laid out. You were asked to consider whether you want quitting forever and whether you should go to twelve-step groups. The experience of twelve-step sobriety and relapse prevention was compared. I talked about how people are often not ready for how alcohol and drugs will leave them wanting them again. What happened to you was explained as a natural response to trying alcohol and drugs. You were given the opportunity to survey some of the impacts alcohol or drug use had on your life, without trying to determine if you were an addict or an alcoholic.

I was explicit with my instructions about how to start thinking about quitting forever through how to carry it out. How to contemplate thoughts of quitting forever were presented, and you were introduced to your ambivalence about alcohol and drug use. How to make up you mind and resolve ambivalence were discussed. The basics of quitting forever were reviewed. Disease concepts were questioned. The natural brain chemistry change and reinforcement qualities of alcohol and drugs were shown as an alternative explanation to disease. You already knew you would think and feel like drinking or using again, and it was explained why you will again feel like drinking or using even after quitting forever. A brain-recovery model was reviewed to show why using alcohol and drugs are always voluntary. The importance of a decision as a starting place was presented as an anchoring point. Choice was compared to a decision. You were given many questions to consider your readiness to change what you are doing by quitting forever.

# Natural Process of Quitting Forever

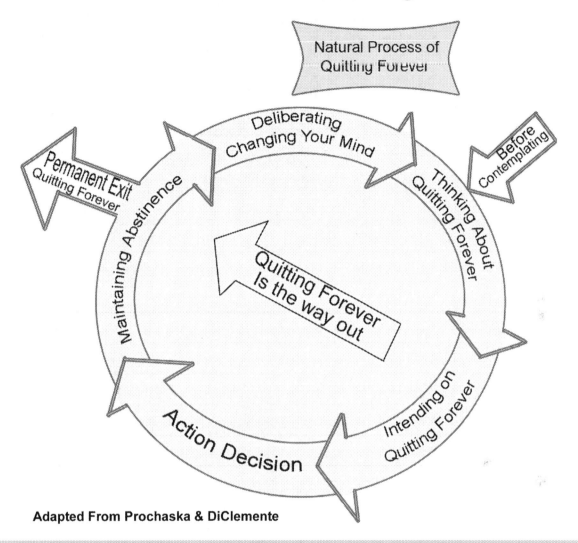

Natural Process of
Quitting Forever

Before
Contemplating

Deliberating
Changing Your Mind

Thinking About
Quitting Forever

Permanent Exit
Quitting Forever

Maintaining Abstinence

Quitting Forever
Is the way out

Intending on
Quitting Forever

Action Decision

**Adapted From Prochaska & DiClemente**

Before contemplating quitting forever, you drank or used drugs as an experiment, got used to the pleasure they bring, and fit them into your lifestyle. You didn't consider quitting forever. For different reasons, you started thinking about quitting forever. The perils of drinking or drugs made you reflect on the notion of change. You were ambivalent in your thinking, wanting to drink and drug and wanting to quit, and you went back and forth between the two ideas. You considered options and made choices alternating between abstaining, controlled drinking and drugging, and sometimes returning to heavy or frequent use. As you resolved your ambivalence, you started intending to quit forever. You may have doubts about your ability to quit forever, but quitting moved into your aim. You developed a purpose to carry out, even if you did not have a design about what to do. Your intention was to quit forever. At some point, you took action. You said to yourself or someone else that you would not drink or drug. Your inclination to carry out the action was determined. You might have carried it out by continuing to make a choice each time you felt like drinking or using. Others made an action decision. Nevertheless, you realized abstaining was for you and you initiated it into action. By not drinking or using, you were maintaining abstinence. When the opportunity to drink or use presented itself, you returned to deliberating your ambivalence and made your choice not to drink or use again. Others who made a decision did not deliberate which choice to make. They were aware of the experience of an urge. They knew that they were going to abstain when they felt the impulse. They used a skill to abstain. Deliberating can be the process of a changing mind. A changing mind goes back and forth ambivalently deliberating what to do. Deliberating carries the risk of drinking or using. Those who do not deliberate and always know what they will do make a permanent exit by quitting forever alcohol and drug use. Permanent exit means you quit forever. You refuse to get caught up in deliberation anymore, because you don't get caught up in your thoughts.

Next, the natural process of quitting forever will be shown. What I am talking about is pragmatic absolutes. There are limited choices in the world. You will either stop using alcohol and drugs or you will use them again. There is no other alternative. The real question is for how long you will stop using alcohol and/or drugs.

# The Model of Quitting Forever

The model of Quitting Forever takes into account both not using and using again. The different parts of the model are not stages because you may see yourself in more than one spot in the model at the same time. For instance, you may maintain abstinence while you deliberate when you should drink again. You may be deliberating whether you should drink again while you intend on quitting forever, or even while you take action and make a decision about quitting forever. You will be shown a way to determine when you have completed quitting forever and made a permanent exit from further alcohol or drug use. You can keep going round and round in a circle, but there is a way out at any time. Quitting forever is the way out.

## Think About Quitting Forever Alcohol and Drug Use

A way to think about quitting alcohol and drugs forever is to begin to contemplate the idea. Contemplate means you are going to consider the idea of permanent, self-decided abstinence. If you have hope of quitting forever, keep your hope. You can make your hope become an action that changes your life forever.

Do not make quitting forever your aim yet if you are not sure what to do. In your consideration, you are not trying to talk yourself into quitting forever. When I say do not aim, I mean I do not want you to direct a course of thinking toward any outcome or result you are committed to pursue if you are not ready. I am not talking about doing something you are not ready to do. If you are ready, skip ahead to "Intend on Quitting Forever."

What you are doing is exploring your ambivalence. If you only wanted to quit forever, you would be determined to begin opposing alcohol and drug use when you felt like drinking or using. You may be abstaining now and already resisting the thought and feelings to use. Have you really thought it out and come to a conclusion you have resolved? Here is a chance to examine your thoughts and feelings in all directions. What are your values? Why would it be important to keep drinking and drugging versus quitting forever?

When contemplating, you are not trying to resolve anything. Contemplation is considering all your thoughts and feelings about the eventual use or quitting of alcohol and drugs. Contemplate by taking any idea that comes to mind and bringing it to a probable end conclusion.

For instance, "I think of using drugs again, and I think of all the fun times with my friends. That idea came to mind. Now I ask myself, what does that do for me? If I continue to use and have fun times with my friends, what will happen as the result of doing that? If I do that again and again, what will happen?" Use your imagination and really ponder with prolonged thinking about the matter. Suppose as many different outcomes you can reason or imagine. Use if-then logic. If "this" happens, then as a result or outcome, "that" will happen. The result or outcome has different possibilities. What is the most likely possible outcome? Contemplation is a willingness to look at the risk of what might happen.

Use your ability to reflect on ideas when you are contemplating. Right now, you may not know if you will abstain or use. It is time to reflect on your thoughts and feelings about drinking and using. You want to reflect on: (1) your reasons to continue, (2) the risks and consequences of drinking and using, and (3) the idea of never using alcohol or drugs again for the remainder of your life. If you can't even think about quitting forever, how will you ever be able to carry it out? Remember, you do not have to make any plans or promises to yourself at this time. It is time to show your willingness to accept how you feel with what you think about quitting forever.

Think quietly and calmly when you reflect. Collect as many ideas and sensations as you experience and really ponder them. Examine ideas attentively and deliberately, and carefully weigh ideas when you ponder. It may be helpful to write your ideas on paper or have someone help you keep a record of them. The purpose of keeping track of your ideas about drinking and/or using versus abstaining is to prevent ruminating. When you ruminate, you go over the same matter again and again with little purposeful thinking. The purpose of contemplation is to think things through by pondering outcomes. It starts with a willingness to accept some discomfort when thoughts come into your awareness.

Some people like to do a cost-benefit analysis when they keep track of their contemplation. Go back to the previous example, "I think of using drugs again, and I think of all the fun times with my friends." Write the idea on a piece of paper. Below the idea, on the right-hand side of the paper, write costs; on the left-hand side, write benefits. Ask yourself, "What are the costs to my family and me if I continue to use drugs or alcohol to have fun times with my friends? What are the benefits?" Guess and suppose as many costs and benefits as you are able to imagine. You can keep adding new thoughts about drinking and drugging to your list or perform a cost-benefit analysis on one of the ideas from the list. One way to add to the list is to take an idea and ask yourself, "What are the costs and benefits of quitting forever?"

Cost-benefit analysis may work for some, but it can be a trap for others. Some people get stuck doing a cost-benefit analysis, because they end up trying to control their thoughts and feelings.

They created a rule that there must be more and better reasons to use than to abstain. However, more reasons to abstain may just create more reasons to use, which now have to be overcome. Now, thoughts and feelings that were supposed to solve the problem have become part of the problem. The real problem may be you are avoiding the experience of how you feel when thinking about quitting forever. What words go though your mind when you think about quitting forever? Write them down, or have someone write them down as they come to you. Examine each thought for what it does for you instead of what it says to you.

Suppose someone else was saying to you the things you wrote down. What would that person be trying to get you to do? If you try to avoid these thoughts you are likely to have them return more often, and they will have more control over you. What are these thoughts doing for you? These thoughts have been added to your experience. They will not go away, because learning works by addition and not subtraction. Something you learned will always be in your mind in some form or anther. You cannot make them go away permanently, although you may not always be mindful of them. It is not bad when you have them, so there is no reason to avoid these thoughts. How do you get untangled from them so they do not keep you stuck?

Fear may be keeping you from thinking about quitting forever. You are taking the words and feelings inside you too literally. Remember, a thought is just a thought, and a feeling is just a feeling. They are both inside you and undetectable to others. Your cost-benefit analysis may be a way you justify your own behavior. Reasons may be helping you avoid what is going on in your life right now in terms of using alcohol or drugs. You may be trapped, avoiding the anxiety that comes along with thinking about quitting forever. You may be evaluating your self negatively when you feel that anxiety, though it is understandable and normal to feel some anxiety when thinking about quitting forever. Your reasons may be influenced by your negative reaction to the thought of quitting forever. People believe their own reasons and become deadlocked in their decision by using reasons to figure out quitting forever.

Do you recognize any ambivalence? Look for how you are simultaneously attracted and repelled by alcohol and drug use. You may fluctuate and go back and forth between the two opposing ideas of drinking and abstaining. When you are ambivalent, you are uncertain which action to follow. Would it be better to go after the benefits and ignore the costs, or avoid the costs and go after the benefits? We are just talking about drinking alcohol or using drugs. Is it worth experimenting, where you try to minimize the costs with controlled drinking or drug use to reduce their harm? Or, is it too big a risk? How many times have you already tried to minimize the costs of continued drinking or drugging by controlling how much or how often you drank or used drugs? Did you try to voluntarily surrender your right to drive while you were drunk or high? Ask yourself, "How important is my getting drunk or high? What makes it so important to me?"

Keep contemplating until it seems like you are going over the same thing again. Ask yourself, "How many times do I need to repeat thinking about the things that happen when I drink or use? Don't I have enough personal experience drinking and/or using drugs to know what is likely to eventually happen? What is more important: words in my head or my direct experience? When will I face what my future intentions are going to be in terms of drinking alcohol or using drugs? How long do I want to put off my personal responsibility to resolve my ambivalence and say what

I want to do the next time I feel like drinking or using or have the opportunity to drink alcohol or use drugs? Why do I have to leave what I will do as a mystery? When will I take responsibility for what I will do when it comes to the possibility of using drugs or drinking alcohol again? What am I doing with my life? What is my intention for the future use of alcohol and drugs? What do I want to happen?"

What have you already tried and how has it worked for you? If you keep doing the same thing, you may be like a person who fell into a deep hole who is trying to dig his/her way out.

Do you have hope of quitting alcohol and drugs forever? You have to do something to get what you are hoping for. Quitting forever is not out of your reach or ability. Just because you continue to have a desire to use does not mean that you cannot quit forever and watch that desire go away over time. You have changed your brain by using alcohol and/or drugs. It will change back as the result of not using, but you have to stop using first. If you want your brain to return to its normal state, never using alcohol or drugs again will get you there. If you have the hope of ending the problems drinking alcohol or using drugs caused, you can turn your hope into intention. Intention is something you are going to do. Don't give up hope. Act on your hope. Your hope will lead you to your values. What you do is your values.

## Intend on Quitting Forever

If it seems likely you are going over the same ideas again and again when you contemplate, it may be time to explore you intentions. You are either going to seek out using alcohol and drugs for your personal pleasure, or you are going to quit and give it up forever. Instead of seeking out alcohol and/or drugs, you may just want to wait to see what you will do when you feel like using or when presented with the opportunity to use. If you are waiting to find out, you are not taking responsibility for your future use. What does your intuition tell you to do?

When I ask you to use your intuition, I am not asking you to do anything more than search for an answer inside you without knowing exactly how you came to the answer. What seems like the right thing for you to do? Don't give reasons, just ask yourself, "What is the thing for me to do?" If the answer is drink or use drugs, ask yourself, "Am I ready to take the responsibility for my actions if I get in trouble using alcohol or drugs again?" If you are ready to take the responsibility, then you are ready to drink and use drugs again, and no one can stop you. You are intending on using alcohol and/or drugs again. It is just a matter of time before you are loaded again. Or, are those just words in your mind. Rely on your experience when using your intuition. We all have to make decisions with incomplete information. You have enough information to figure out what you determine is best for you.

Other people are able reason with themselves and resolve their intention. Reason is when you use rational thinking and tell yourself what is the best thing to do. Resolve is when you take your ambivalence about thinking both ways and decide which side you will be on. You can only be on the side of using again or quitting forever. It is just one way or the other, not both ways. What does your experience tell you about which side will be in-line with your values?

You can see yourself thinking about both drinking/using drugs and quitting forever. After careful consideration, quitting forever is the thing for you to do. In your mind, you can still hear the other side, which wants to drink or drug. But, you know that is not the thing for you to do anymore. The thing for you to do is to quit forever. At that point, you have an intention about quitting forever. If you have intention about quitting forever, your values are changing.

If you do not want to risk getting loaded again with the difficulties drinking and drugging bring, then it is likely time for you to declare your intentions to yourself. Are you going to continue choosing whether you will drink and/or drug, or are you going to start intending to make a decision about quitting forever? What would you do with your life if you never drank or drugged again? What would you have done with your life if you had already finished quitting forever?

Intending is a state of mind about what is to be done. Is your purpose to quit forever, even though you have not yet done it? Quitting forever is something you will bring about once you have the intention of quitting forever. Intention often comes out of recognizing and dealing with or resolving ambivalence.

When you were ambivalent, you were thinking about using and not using again, and you were going back and forth. Now, you are resolved to not using again, ever. You made up your mind to follow your values and never drink or use drugs again. When your mind goes back and forth and you observe what your mind is doing and willingly accept your internal experience, let it be mind chatter and follow your values based on your own personal experience.

Right now, the decision facing you is whether you are quitting alcohol and drugs forever. It is time to arrive at a solution to end the uncertainty of what you will do. In your judgment, should you be quitting alcohol or drugs forever? You may not be ready to say when you will be quitting forever, but are you ready to end your uncertainty about whether quitting forever is the thing for you to do. What is the right thing to do? What is important to you?

When you tell yourself that quitting forever is the thing for you to do, you have the intention to quit forever. Quitting forever is something you will do. It may be just a wish or a need right now, but the intention of quitting forever exists. Quitting forever is something you will bring about now that you are intending on quitting. You're in a state of mind that the act of quitting forever is the thing you will eventually make happen. If you are still choosing, your state of mind switches back and forth. With a decision, you know where you will settle your mind if you feel it switch back and forth. As soon as your mind starts switching back and forth in a return of ambivalent deliberation, you can rely on your decision. Ask yourself, "Why am I going over this issue again? I already decided I will quit. Is there something more to figure out?" If you have new information to consider, then return to contemplating, reflect on the new information, ponder outcomes, and review what is the best thing for you to do. If the information is not new, are you ruminating over the same ideas again and again? When is it time to start relying on your decided intent? You can follow your values when words in your mind do not agree. When will you start acting on your values?

At times, you may still think about a return to drinking or drugging. Some people will tell you a notion about drinking or using is a lapse. A lapse is an interruption for a period of time. A lapse is temporary deviation in thinking from your intention to quit forever. It is natural for your mind to go back and forth between the two ideas. Have you bought into the thought about drinking or using? Remember, the thought is not an action. A notion to drink or use drugs is your past experience that either popped into your head, you became aware of the feeling, or you chose to think about using again. You know the experience is a whim, because it is a sudden idea that is a change of mind, direction, and value. What will it do for you if you act on this whim?

You know you decided to quit forever. Will you treat this notion to use as a fancy or a caprice? They are just words in your mind passing through. Have you returned to contemplating whether or not to quit. Ask yourself if you are re-deciding or has the idea just popped into your mind with feeling to carry it out? An idea that suddenly appears is not to be heeded, because past use of alcohol or drugs can make you feel impulsive. Recognize that idea for what it is, a whim or a notion going against your intention to quit forever. You can treat the notion as a caprice or a notion that was unmotivated and maybe unpredictable. Do not return to pondering the use of alcohol or drugs, or you will be going backward. You can re-anchor your decision to act on your values by saying to yourself, "I know I will be quitting forever. This notion to drink or use again is mind chatter. I am quitting forever, no matter what my mind tells me. My experience tells me it is the thing to do. Isn't it interesting to observe the mind recovering from alcohol and drugs."

Now that you have decided that quitting forever is the thing to do, what you want to be pondering is, "When will I carry out the decision to quit forever?" You may want to daydream about a time when your drinking and drugging days are over. In your imagination, can you imagine never drinking or drugging again? Think about how you would carry it out. When and how would you put that into action? Will you follow your values or your mind chatter?

## Action Decision

Some people have the intent to quitting forever but never take the necessary action. Here are a few reasons that get stuck in their minds:

1. Twelve-step groups and substance abuse counselors discourage people from quitting forever when they hawk their one-day-at-a-time motto.

2. When someone talks about the intention to quit forever, he or she have heard discouraging recovery slogans like, "Never say never," and "The road to hell is paved with good intentions," or a favorite *Big Book* slogan, "Your best thinking got you here."

3. Counting time gone without drinking gets you looking in the wrong direction. People say, "I have gone ninety days without drinking. I am not currently drinking. I don't have a plan to drink at this time." Having no plan to drink is not the same as having a plan not to drink. Counting time without drinking or using is looking at the past. A decision to never drink or drug again is looking at now and the future.

4. The idea that disease makes you drink leaves some people unsure if they have the ability to quit forever. They learned they relapse and something out of their control

will happen. They were told trying to abstain from alcohol or drugs was like having diarrhea. You can hold out for a while but you can't help it when it happens. It is not your fault when you drink or use drugs because you have a disease.

5. Some people have tried to quit forever but went back to drinking and drugging. Because they didn't do it, they now believe they cannot do it. Why would you promise yourself something you do not think you have the ability to carry out?

6. If someone believes they are an alcoholic or an addict, they come to think that is why they carry out the behavior. People who call themselves alcoholic or addict often use those labels to explain why they drink or drug. How could an addict ever promise himself or herself they would never use again? They have been told, "Once an alcoholic or an addict, always an alcoholic or addict." If that is what you are, how can you stop being what you are?

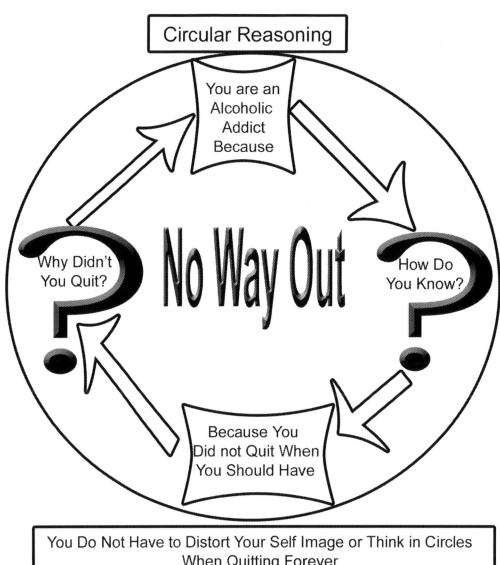

7. People were told they have to work through all their issues before they can quit. You have problems that make you drink or drug. Without first solving those problems, you cannot keep yourself from drinking or drugging. Don't say you won't drink/drug until you have worked out all your issues.

8. Other people intend to quit forever but put off the action decision and never make the action decision. They just don't drink or drug for a while and forget about the idea of quitting forever. Then, after a time of not drinking or drugging, they start up again for various reasons. They then say, "I don't understand why I started drinking/drugging again after I quit." The answer is that they never quit forever; they just stopped. If they did say to themselves that they quit forever, then they changed their mind. They did not know how to use the skill of quitting forever.

The following is a rational review of each reason that gets stuck in the mind.

## One Day at a Time

There is no evidence that only quitting one day at a time is better than quitting forever. There is plenty of anecdotal evidence that quitting forever not only works better than tentative one day at a time but is also the natural thing to do. Many of us know someone who used to drink and drug, but who no longer does and quit without any help from the twelve steps or recovery counselors. Ask them how they did it. Usually, they cannot give too much detail other than that they just quit. Sticking with one day at a time is giving up hope you to will someday quit forever.

*Living one day at a time;*
*enjoying one moment at a time;*
*accepting hardships as the pathway to peace;*
*http://www.aahistory.com/prayer.html*

The motto "one day at a time" was taken from the Serenity Prayer. Dr. Rheinhold Niebuhr wrote the prayer for World War II troops. The earliest reference to the phrase is from the Roman philosopher Cicero. The Serenity Prayer reads, "Living life one day at a time," and does not say to only quit alcohol one day at a time. One day at a time may be good advice on how to practice mindfulness and focus on the moment, but it is not about avoiding responsible plans for the future.

The counseling wisdom behind one-day-at-a-time quitting advice is if you commit for one day, then you will not be disappointed when you relapse. Why set yourself up for failure by promising something you cannot carry out? If you say you won't drink or drug anymore and you get loaded again, you will feel so bad about yourself that it will make things worse. Just go one day at a time until it gets easier. See if you can just stay sober for today.

Quitting one day at a time may be a way to start for some people, but it is very limiting in that you can never go on to quitting forever. If you can keep yourself from drinking and drugging for one day, that proves you can keep yourself from drinking and drugging. Why should you be forced into limiting your commitment to one day? One-day-at-a-time recovery keeps you from resolving the question, "Am I going to drink alcohol or use drugs anymore?" One day at a time means one is hopeless about ever answering that question.

Now that you have been clean and sober for a number of days, what is your plan for the future use of alcohol or drugs? If you intend on quitting forever, when will you carry out the intent? If you feel unsure about quitting forever, is it a plan to drink or use again? Ask yourself if you want to carry out a plan to use alcohol and drugs again, or if you want to forever end the use. Plenty of people don't use again when they feel like using by focusing on the future, a time when they will not feel like using because they did not use when they felt like using in the present. It won't always feel like this. I am willing to accept how I feel right now because I know I will never pick up alcohol or drugs because of the way I feel.

## Never Say Never

The phrase, "never say never," is not only poor advice, it is self-contradictory. Recognize the self-contradiction in the phrase. If I commit to never saying never, I am actually saying never. Following out the advice of the phrase goes against the advice of the phrase. It is easy to carry out the advice of never saying never, because saying never is such a common thing for people to do. Saying you will never again do something that you want to end is an expression of hope and intent. Never say never is a phrase easy to remember, but it is certainly not a guiding principle to follow when talking about voluntary behavior.

Ordinary people have plenty of things they say to themselves they will never do like robbery, murder, and molest, gross things most people say they will never do, and most people carry out their pledge. When people get married, they say forever, never to part. Even if they get divorced, many remarry forever and never get divorced again. Others get divorced and say they will never marry again and live the remainder of their lives as single people. The examples of people saying never and carrying out never for the remainder of their lives could fill a book. Think about some of the things you did at a younger age that you now know you will never do again, and you will get an idea of how common it is to say never again and carry it out. You realize it is time to do things differently. You hope you can change. You make the change and never do what they quit again. Never doing something again that you once enjoyed, while remembering the pleasure you felt doing it is a common experience.

## Counting Time

Counselors and the twelve-step movement encourage you to count time sober. The premise is people who are sober longer are doing better. The support group can give you encouragement for not drinking and/or drugging. If you are in a twelve-step group, not drinking means you are working a good program. Being sober for a period of time means you are receiving divine guidance from your supernatural higher power or your God. You can get a chip for further reinforcement and to show your family and friends how good you are doing. If you are using relapse-prevention skills, it means you are making the right choices and avoiding apparently irrelevant choices. If you drink or use drugs, you lose your time sober and start back at zero.

The problem with counting time is it keeps you focused on how long you have gone without. Counting time sober can be a way to tell when it is time to use again. Generally, we keep track of time doing without as a way to determine if it is time to indulge and drink or use drugs. "Who can really blame me for doing it again after all the time I went without?"

Question the relevancy of counting time. Why bother to count time if you are never going to use again? What does it do for you? If you say it helps you know that you have really quit forever, then you have not quit forever. Knowing you have quit forever is not dependent on how long you have not drank or used drugs. Knowing you have quit forever is a subjective feeling you have after not drinking or drugging when the opportunity presents. If you are 100 percent sure you will never drink or drug again after drinking and drugging places have come and gone, then you probably have quit forever.

What does counting time do for you if you are never going to use again? There is no evidence people who count the time not drinking or drugging abstain longer than those who don't count time. Quitting forever is not about how long you have not used alcohol or drugs, but how long you will not use alcohol or drugs. If it is difficult to talk about how long you are not going to use alcohol or drugs, you are facing your feeling to use again. Facing the feeling to use again is part of quitting alcohol or drugs. Counting time takes you in the opposite direction of how long you will not use alcohol or drugs. Counting time means reviewing what you have done and not facing your responsibility of what you will do. Quitting forever means the length of time you have not used no longer matters to you because it is forever. Forever means you will never again drink alcohol or use drugs for any reason. It makes counting time irrelevant.

## Disease Concept of Addiction

Alcohol and drug use cause disease, but a disease does not cause alcohol and drug use. There are some problems with calling alcohol and drug use a disease. It confuses cause with effect. It presents a model, or concept, for understanding what has happened to you and makes it seem like the act of consuming alcohol or drugs is an actual affliction. Saying a disease causes you to drink alcohol or use drugs makes it sound like using is a passive action that just happens by itself. The biological explanations showing how alcohol and drug addiction are diseases leave out an important part of how your voluntary biology takes place. Disease explanations lead you to a different solution than to quit forever. Believing you have a disease that makes you use alcohol or drugs keeps you from fully recovering because the disease is a chronic condition.

Let us think about the diseases of alcoholism and drug addiction. How does a disease make you put alcohol or drugs in your body when you do not want them there? Those who preach the disease concept state that alcohol and drug use start out as voluntary actions. Brain scan pictures are used to show brain changes in people with extreme heavy alcohol or drug use. Has anyone done a brain scan on you to show your brain has changed so much that you cannot keep yourself from drinking or using? It is a fact: the brain changes as the result of drug use. The fact reemphasizes the mix-up in cause and effect. Using alcohol and/or drugs caused the brain change; the brain change did not cause the use of alcohol or drugs. Where is the evidence that your brain has changed enough that you cannot keep yourself from using again?

## You Believe You Cannot Quit Forever

You said you would not drink or use drugs, and then you went and drank or used drugs again. Not doing what you intended to do does not mean you are unable. If not being able to do something you tried to do meant you could not do it, then no one could ever learn to do something once they tried and did not succeed. It would also mean people who tried again would never be able to do what they wanted. Saying you cannot do something when you did not do something is like giving yourself a pass-fail test. If you fail, you tell yourself you cannot succeed. You give up hope and give up learning.

If you tried to quit and did not quit, you may be holding something against yourself that will never change. You said you would not use, then you went and used. That act of using cannot be undone. If you hold that against yourself, you have given yourself a life sentence of failure. If you are detoxed right now, drinking and drugging is in the past, it is something that is unchangeable. Where is it that was the proof you can never quit now or in the future when you quit again? If you cannot do something and get new information about how to do it, then what you learned can help you to act differently when you apply the new information. Remember how your brain and body works together. Who controls your hands?

Perhaps you said you would never use again, and you were unprepared for the desire that primitive part of your brain can produce to get what it wants. Alcohol and drugs really do give you an appetite to use them again. Unless you have a plan for what to do when that appetite presents itself, you may not have the skill to keep a fixed decision when you feel like drinking or using drugs. If your mind was not completely made up, you likely started deliberating whether you should drink or use when you felt strongly like doing it. It was really easy to change your mind.

When you said you wouldn't use again, did you really think it through, or did you say it in desperation after some uncomfortable event brought on by drinking or drug use? It is not uncommon for someone to wake up with a hangover and say never again, only to drink that very afternoon. Saying never again as a snap answer to your problem is different than really thinking it through and saying to yourself you will never drink or drug again. When you say it in a snap decision, you have no intention of not changing your mind. You had not made a fixed decision and were likely choosing. Although, we now know that many people just quit without thinking much about it. Some people just quit forever without going into reasons why they should. They quit and never using again because they quit forever and it had meaning for them as a value.

Many people who have said they quit forever, never sat down and thought about what forever means to them. If you stop for a while but have no intention of quitting forever, it is understandable why you would drink alcohol or use drugs again. Your concept of forever was never really defined. Even though you said the word "forever" to yourself, it may not have meant for the remainder of your life. Other people who really did mean forever were faced with the idea of just one more time. They quit forever, but did not say goodbye to the high. It was easy to give in to just one more time, but now you have given in to just one more time many times and doubt your ability to quit forever.

You may have quit conditionally. Conditional quitting is when you say that your life will be better after you quit alcohol or drugs, then something unfortunate happens like a death in the family or the end of a relationship. You say to yourself, "I never meant I would not drink or drug under these conditions," and you go back on your word to yourself. That means you did not quit forever. It does not mean that you cannot quit forever. Unconditional quitting is when you quit no matter what happens in your life. You have a fixed decision and do not change your mind based on the situation.

Go back and review the process of quitting forever diagram. You are just maintaining sobriety until quitting forever. If you are maintaining, then you have not quit forever. You want to understand the brain-recovery model and how to make a fixed decision. You want to learn how to separate from the feeling to use. You want to learn to take an aggressive stance based on a decision to not drink or use rather than a defensive stance left up to choice.

People are quitting forever, and you are no different if you want to quit using alcohol and drugs. Your body is fully capable of controlling your hands. Your desire to drink alcohol or use drugs cannot move your hands unless you want them to move and pick up drinks or drugs. Just because you did not does not mean you cannot. Do not give up hope and hold your past against yourself. You have new information: quitting forever. You can make a decision and stop waiting and fighting your thoughts and feelings. Full recovery is within your grasp. Quit and quit again until it is forever.

## You Believe You Are an Alcoholic or an Addict

Saying you are an alcoholic or an addict is assuming a deviant role identity. Becoming an alcoholic or addict can become a reason to drink or use again. People who call themselves alcoholic or addict are doing something that has nothing to do with quitting forever.

Alcoholic and addict as identity labels are as self concept not to be proud of. Except when the importance is distorted by a recovery group, very few people want to identify themselves this way and feel good about it. You don't take on the label of other problems. The idea of role recovery comes from rehabilitation. In rehabilitation, people are encouraged not to think of themselves as a negative label and are instead encouraged to recover their perception of themselves as an ordinary label. Why can't you just assume a positive role of mother, father, sister, or brother? What is wrong with just being who you are and going by your name like you do elsewhere? Except when joining a twelve-step group, calling yourself alcoholic or addict has little value and has nothing to do with whether you decide to quit forever. We don't want to erase the stigma of being an alcoholic or addict. It would be better to not act like one and to assume the identity of one who never drinks or drugs.

Calling yourself an alcoholic or addict is circular reasoning. As the logic goes, you know you are an alcoholic or addict because you kept drinking and or using when you would have been better off quitting. And, why didn't you quit? You did not quit because you are an alcoholic or addict. Using a label to explain a behavior, while using the behavior to justify the label, is clearly circular reasoning. Studies have shown that people who refuse to call themselves alcoholic or addict do no worse and sometimes do better at recovery than people who identify themselves with the label.

People who call themselves alcoholic or addict sometimes use the label as a reason why they keep drinking and drugging. "I relapsed because I am an alcoholic." Don't you know that is what drug addicts do? When you believe that is what you are, it closes the door to being something different. What you have done is turned a verb into a noun. A verb is an action word. Drink is a verb. Drink is an action or behavior. When you label yourself as your behavior, you make it more difficult to change that behavior because of the way you think about it. For example, wave your arm. Did that make your identity an arm waver? It is silly to think you are any behavior you do, even if you do them again and again. Are you still an arm waver when you are not waving your arm?

Many people say they are never going to drink alcohol or use drugs again, because they do not want to be an alcoholic or addict. That may make some sense, but it makes absolutely no sense to quit drinking and drugging and still call yourself an alcoholic or addict. The question is why do you have to call yourself an alcoholic or addict in order to quit? You really don't have to call yourself any pejorative names. If you have a reason for quitting and intend on quitting forever, you can call yourself your own name and be anything you want. You have plenty of positive role names to call yourself. If you are going to be anything, be something you can be proud of.

## Solve Problems First or Quit Forever to Solve Problems

The idea you have to solve problems before you can quit forever is the psychological-disease concept. The assumption that a problem makes someone drink or use drugs is faulty. How can a problem make you move your arms to pick up alcohol or drugs when you do not want to pick them up? Problems cannot force you to drink or use drugs. Many counselors say problems are what makes you want to use alcohol or drugs.

Reconsider if a problem makes you want to use alcohol or drugs. Begin by pondering whether when you have a problem, if you use any drug or just your favorite one. Someone who likes to drink alcohol will go and get drunk when they have a problem. Most people who get drunk will not go shoot heroin when they have a problem. If a problem makes you use, why doesn't it make you use all drugs? The answer is because you have to have used the drug and liked the high. You are not running from a problem, but you are running to the high. You don't run to a high that you have not fallen in love with. Someone who loves heroin will not go and shoot speed when they have a problem; they will shoot heroin. When you have a problem, you know that you can be drunk or high instead of feeling unhappy about your problem, so you go after the high. You could be solving the problem while you accept you might have a life event that is sad to experience while not drinking or using drugs.

While high, you still know you have a problem, but you feel loaded. Someone who is high on alcohol or a drug will even think about ways to solve the problem. Trying to solve problems while high is very inefficient and often prevents you from solving the problem. Even if you come up with a solution, you are less likely to persist and carry out the solution, because solving problems often means persisting and working to perfect an imperfect solution until you find a better way.

Only an alcohol or drug problem can be solved immediately. During the first minute of quitting forever, your alcohol and/or drug problem is forever solved. The effects of using alcohol or drugs may have left you with some problems to solve, but after you quit forever, doing things you regret while you are drunk or high will be over.

Now that you never drink alcohol or use drugs, what problem do you want to work at solving? You don't solve the problem to keep yourself from using alcohol or drugs. You now solve the problem just for the solution. For example, a therapist might have you work on your anger toward your husband or wife so that you do not drink or use drugs anymore. After quitting forever, you work on your anger toward your husband or wife to have a better relationship with that person. And, when your relationship does not get better quickly, you keep working on the problem rather than go out and drink or use drugs. You quit using alcohol or drugs to solve problems. You don't solve problems to quit using alcohol or drugs.

Furthermore, if you are solving problems to quit using alcohol or drugs, the therapist tells you which problem to work on, because they found the problem that makes you use. After quitting forever, you are the one to pick which problem to solve. Solve any, all, or none of your problems. Choose with whom you wish to solve your problems. I solve problems using cognitive behavioral therapy and was trained in Rational Emotive Behavioral Therapy by Albert Ellis. Some people would rather work with a Freudian psychoanalyst, get nondirective therapy, or work with a priest, minister, or rabbi. Other people like to solve problems on their own, using friends and family. Self-help books are another popular way to solve problems, although many self-help books will often take you back to the twelve steps.

After quitting forever, you decide what problem to work on, how you are going to solve the problem, and who you want to work with to solve the problem. You solve the problem for the solution, not to keep yourself from using. What do you want to do with your life once you never use alcohol or drugs again? Not using alcohol or drugs will solve some of life's problems and leave you open to a new way of living. How are you going to live your life now that you never use alcohol or drugs?

## Putting Off Quitting Forever: Procrastination

Just because you decided quitting forever is the thing to do, it does not mean you have done it. Quitting forever is an event that takes place in your life. Quitting forever is something you have done. Once you have quit forever, the act is over and you are finished. If you do not believe you are finished, then either you have not completed quitting forever or that after quitting forever, you have doubts about carrying it out.

If you intend to quit forever and have not, ask yourself, "When am I quitting forever?" It is time to answer that question. You can tell yourself when because that is how it gets done. Pick a date and a time. Say to yourself, "After that day and time, I will *never* use alcohol or drugs again." Never is the way to talk to yourself, because you spent a lot of time contemplating and talking to yourself about why you should be quitting forever. It is time to end the talk of reasons and get on with quitting forever, so you can move away from reasons to drink or not to drink.

After quitting forever, you will use just one reason: because you have done it. Quitting forever means that you have reviewed the reasons long enough and want to bring that part, along with your drinking or drug use, to a conclusion. You will now only use one reason to stand for all those reasons you considered. The reason you don't drink or drug is because you made a decision about quitting forever. The decision is, "I will never pick up alcohol or drugs again with my hands to put them into my body. I have the ability to control my hands and arms. I don't have to keep going over a lot of reasons not to drink or use drugs anymore. I don't have to run from my thoughts and feelings to drink or drug, and I don't have to fight them."

If you are putting off quitting forever, are procrastinating. Procrastinating is a word meaning to put off something intentionally, something you know you should do. If you hear words your mind, "How do I know I intend on quitting forever?" Then, go back and read the section on intending to quit. Do you know the moral reason for quitting forever? Why are you putting off the decision? Do you want another round of drinking or drug use? Ask yourself, "How long will I keep doing this? How many more times will I do it again?" If you do not have an immediate, short, action answer that you can carry out, you may be caught up in mind chatter spending time thinking what to do when thinking about what to do is keeping you from doing.

Saying, "I know I should quit forever, but I am not ready right now," is a plan to drink or use drugs again. Why are you not ready if you are not going to drink or drug again? You would only be not ready if you wanted to have a chance at drinking or drugging again. People who have not quit but who are putting off quitting forever usually say, "But I am not thinking about drinking or drugging and haven't been doing it." Saying you are not thinking about it and not drinking or drugging is like saying why fix the roof when it isn't leaking. The roof isn't leaking because it is not raining. When it is raining, you can't fix the roof until it is dry. When it is dry, why bother to fix the roof because it is not leaking. Let me state the roof analogy more literally in the terms of alcohol or drug use. "Why should I be quitting forever? I am not drinking or using drugs, and I do not feel like drinking or using drugs. If I drink or use drugs, it will be too late for quitting, but I don't think that will happen. If it doesn't happen, then I would not need to quit forever. Let's just wait and see what happens." Those are the basic thoughts of procrastination. There are too many unanswered questions. The above thoughts are not well developed and lack depth of self-understanding and self-responsibility.

You can recognize procrastinating thoughts by these three elements:

1. You say you are not doing it and not thinking about doing it.

2. You draw a conclusion: since I am not, then it will not.

3. You use the conclusion as a reason to put off something, reasoning that since it will not happen, it does not have to be done.

Having to wait to see what happens reveals the weakness in your strategy. Waiting to see what happens is passive and inaccurate thinking. There is a difference between what happens and what you will do. What will happen is inevitable. When something is inevitable, you will not be able to avoid or evade it. What is inevitable is you will not be able to avoid being in the presence of alcohol or drugs for the remainder of your life. Alcohol and drugs are there for the purchase and often for the asking. Trying to avoid the presence of alcohol and/or drugs is not worth the gamble. If they are not in your presence, then you don't use them. But, as soon as they are offered, you are at risk of trying them again. You do not know what you are going to do when you are offered the opportunity to drink or drug. It is like living your life in fear or with insecurity.

The second inevitability is you are likely going to feel like drinking alcohol and/or using drugs again. What are you going to do when you are in the presence of alcohol and/or drugs and feel like using alcohol or drugs?

Remember how difficult it was to ponder the idea of quitting forever when you were relaxed and focused? When alcohol or drugs are in reach, and you feel like using them, you may not feel calm and relaxed or focused. You may feel under pressure. The pressure you feel will be that of indecision. You have not decided what to do. You will have a forced choice. Your choice is to pick up alcohol and/or drugs and put them into your body or let them lie there. You don't know what you are going to do ahead of time. You will have to choose what to do. People are looking at you and waiting. If you don't do it, you may miss the chance and be left out. You have an opportunity waiting for you. You have been waiting for this opportunity to find out what you will do. You can't both drink and use drugs and abstain from use at the same time.

Let us wait and see what you will do. It is a safe bet you would find yourself in a scene like this. What you will do (your behavior) in the scene is not yet determined unless you quit forever. When you procrastinate, you wait to find out what you will do. When you put off quitting forever, you hold the door open to drink alcohol and/or use drugs again if you want to when the opportunity or situation presents itself. Once you understand the brain-recovery model, it is easy to understand why you will want to drink or use drugs again because you have drank and used previously, and the feeling to use is an involuntary response from a primitive part of your brain. Your drinking or drugging actions have been reinforced as the substance stimulated your pleasure center. You have been reinforced for going through the voluntary motions of drinking alcohol or using drugs stimulating your pleasure pathways of reward. That is why you will feel like doing it again. That is the hardest time to figure out what to do. If you didn't figure it out when it was easier, why would you think you could figure out what to do when it was harder?

Go over the same scene after quitting forever. Quitting forever means saying to yourself: "I know I will likely be around alcohol and/or drugs again. I know when that happens, I may have the feeling to drink or use drugs. When it happens, I know what I will do because I *never* drink or use under any circumstances. I know I control my hands and arms. I know I quit. I am in control of my arms and hands and know what I am going to do with them. I am not going to pick up alcohol or drugs and put them into my body."

It is a secure feeling to be in control of yourself in this one area. You may not be able to predict when you will be fired from you job or when you will run a stop sign while driving. You may not be able to tell if or when your husband/wife or boy-/girlfriend will leave you. You may not even know if you will ever be homeless. But, you can always be sure of your ability to not pick up what you do not want to pick up. And, you know you will never pick up alcohol or drugs and put them into your body. It is one of the few things of which you can be sure.

Once you have made the decision to never pick up and use alcohol and/or drugs, you are waiting to carry out your decision. Your decision to quit forever is the start. Now you want to go and lead your life like you will never again use alcohol or drugs. You are waiting for alcohol or drugs so you can abstain in their presence. You are waiting for the feeling to drink or use drugs so you can control your hands. The decision is only part of quitting forever. You want to have the experience of using the decision and abstaining when you have the opportunity or feel like drinking or drugging. The decision is the mind part. The experience of carrying out the decision is the behavior part. It is time to practice your skill. How quickly can you recognize an opportunity or feeling and know you will never use? The experience is what you want to talk about at Quitting Forever after you make the decision to quit forever.

## Maintaining Abstinence

Now that you have decided to never drink or use drugs again, it is time to carry out your decision. The decision is only part of quitting forever. To complete quitting forever, you use the decision as a value to abstain. You have to have the experience of refusing to drink alcohol or use drugs. How do you use your decision to abstain? You can use imagination and practice in your mind, carrying out exercises where you willingly let thoughts and feelings to use alcohol and drugs pass through your mind without you catching on to them to follow them while you observe them moving along without meaning of what you will do. You can talk about your experience of what you thought, how you felt, what you did, and what you said to others when you felt like drinking or using. You will abstain in-vivo, meaning in your living sometimes in the presence of alcohol or drugs or while other people drink or use drugs when you do not.

Until you have made a permanent exit, you are just maintaining your abstinence. Abstinence means you voluntarily do not indulge your appetite for alcohol or drugs. Your appetite may be brought on by cues associated with your former using days, or it may happen for no reason.

Observe what goes on when you feel like using alcohol or drugs and when they are in your presence. Are you arguing with yourself? Maintaining abstinence is not the same thing as quitting forever with permanent exit from further alcohol and drug use. Maintaining means your existing state is clean and sober. You are defending your sobriety from a relapse when you maintain abstinence. You persevere in not drinking or drugging by going day by day without drinking. You persevere in talking your way out of drinking or drugging when you have the urge. Maintaining is easy at times and more of a struggle other times. You just don't know what is going to happen or what you will do when it does happen. Maintaining is a state of not being drunk or high on drugs now, but it is also a state of being unsure what you will do in the future. If you are holding onto a period of time without drinking or using drug then you are maintaining abstinence. Maintaining is good enough to watch time pass and avoid getting drunk or high. You might not go someplace you want to go because you are afraid you might drink alcohol or use drugs there.

Why risk it when you are doing so well? But, at the same time, you sometimes feel left out and wish you could go where you want.

Maintaining abstinence means working hard to control your inner self. Thoughts and feelings of using alcohol and drugs must be avoided. You watch for red flags that might trigger your desire to drink or use drugs. If the thoughts persist, you debate them and argue with yourself in a desperate attempt to resist. It may seem like no one knows how hard you are trying. It may feel as though you could use more support. You are controlling yourself and not drinking or drugging. If only someone would appreciate how hard you are trying. Sometimes it is easy not to drink or drug. Other times it is really difficult, especially when the thoughts and feelings to drink or use drugs returns. If you can just make it through those times, you will have it made. Days without drinking or drugging count for you. You watch them go by, adding up as proof to yourself you are doing it.

You look for something to replace alcohol and drug use when you are maintaining. Perhaps you find a hobby or a club to join to occupy your time. You've got to find something worthwhile to keep your mind off drinking alcohol or using drugs. You need to find something to do instead of drinking or drugging.

Drinking or drugging is a choice you have to make. You better make the right choice, or you will be losing time clean and sober. Sometimes you might feel anxious or afraid you might drink or use drugs again. You work hard to distract yourself from that feeling when it happens, because thinking too far ahead can get you in trouble. You just have to stay in control and make the right choices.

You need to find new friends who do not drink or use drugs. Your old friends are not good for you, and you are afraid to be around them because they might ask you to have a drink or use a drug. It is easy to see people divided into two categories: those who do not drink or drug and those who do. The wrong people have to be avoided because of how you might feel if you were around them.

You have to watch how you feel when you are maintaining. If you become too emotional, you might blow it. You better keep your cool. Getting hungry, angry, lonely, or tired could set you off on another bender or runner. Suppose you lose control and started drinking or drugging again?

You need to keep those reasons not to drink or drug fresh in your mind while maintaining. You need to keep going over the bad consequences of drinking or drugging not to lose sight of them. You never know when you are going to have to fight that beast inside you that wants a drink or drug. What if the committee inside your head starts talking to you? You've got to keep in control of what is going on in your mind or it could get out of hand.

You may feel like giving yourself reasons not to drink or drug, but that is not relying on your decision. For example, you are at a party with an open bar, and they bring free drinks to your table and set them in front of you. You realize the drink is within your reach. You really feel like taking a drink. Instead of saying to yourself, "No, I never drink anymore," some people instead say, "This is not a good idea, because I will get in trouble." Not wanting to be in trouble is a good reason not to drink or use drugs, but it is an excuse or a bargain not to drink. Saying you will not drink to avoid trouble sets up the opposite side of the coin: you would drink if you would not get in trouble. Now the bargaining begins. You can start deliberating under what situations you could drink or use drugs and not be in trouble.

## Quitting Forever: Permanent Exit

You have moved on to permanent exit when you are completely confident you will never again use alcohol or drugs. Once you have the experience of feeling like taking a drink or using drugs, you may have the opportunity to use. That experience can move you beyond maintaining abstinence. You can tell if you have made a permanent exit by your experience. You will always abstain when you have the opportunity and the feeling to drink alcohol or use drugs if you know you will never do it because you are 100 percent confident you will carry out abstinence for the remainder of your life while you feel good about abstaining. Quitting forever starts at some point in time in your life. Permanent abstinence has to start at some point in time.

Nobody else can really know about your quitting forever, and you cannot prove it. But, you will know. The remaining thing for you to do at this point is to quit the recovery movement, quit attending Quitting Forever. Stop reading about alcohol and drug recovery, and get on with your life by never drinking alcohol or using drugs. You do not have to live the life as an ex-alcoholic or ex-addict. Just be yourself, and do what you want to do without drinking or drugging.

You might recognize alcohol or drugs are around for you to use. You might find yourself reminded of times when you did drink or use drugs. You might hear an inner voice saying, "Just one more time. Nobody will ever know. Let's have a drink or get high." You might dream about drinking or using. You might catch yourself in a daydream about it. You may experience a desire to drink or use drugs when leaving work or when driving home in your car. Just notice when the experience happens and acknowledge that it happened. Wherever and whenever it happens, you know what you will do. It is always the same, and you get better at it the more you do it. Know you will never drink or use drugs whenever you recognize a thought, feeling, desire, appetite, or opportunity to drink alcohol or use drugs because you control your hands. You can say to yourself, "I quit forever. I never drink or use drugs." It is even better if you don't say it because you already know it and there is nothing to say. You know what you do has more meaning than what you say. You never drink or use drugs. What else is there to say? Now, control your hands and arms, and do not pick up alcohol or drugs to put into your body. You do not have to control your inner experience and stop other thoughts and sensations from being present. Accept them and control your hands.

If you experience anything that supports the idea of drinking or using drugs, it is time to use your skill. Make room for the idea to be present. You don't have to make it go away. It cannot move your hands. Ideas to drink or use are just words in your head—mind chatter. Do not start reasoning or arguing a point. Why would you buy into thinking about situations where you could drink or use drugs after quitting forever?

**Experience Exercise:** Are you ready to try an imaginary exercise to practice your skill? Get comfortable. Feel the chair underneath you and your feet on the floor. Blink, and feel the tongue in your mouth. Focus on your breathing and catch your breath. Let your breathing become calm, easy, and regular. Follow your breathing in and out. What is your decision about the future use of alcohol and drugs? Focus on your feeling to never again drink or use. Anchor to the value and feeling you will never again drink alcohol or use drugs as something you do no a set of words you say. Fix your vision on one thing in front of you. Let your eyes blink until they close.

Now, start the exercise. Imagine your favorite drink or drug right in front of you. See it in your mind. Remember how good it felt. When you can feel the appetite, desire, or a thought to use comes to mind, notice what that feels like. Acknowledge to yourself the change in your mind as it went from not thinking about alcohol and drugs to the experience of thinking about alcohol and drugs. Observe and describe your experience.

Open your eyes. You engaged what caused you to drink alcohol or use drugs in the past. Focus on your decision to never again use. Has your value of quitting forever changed? You know you never again use alcohol or drugs, and what you just experienced is what will happen. You will feel like drinking or using drugs again. Nothing will force you to use alcohol or drugs if you do not want to. The part of your brain that wants it is not the part of our brain that can pick it up. The area in the brain where you made your decision rules the part of your brain that lets you pick of up alcohol or drugs. You cannot pick up alcohol or drugs unless you change your mind. Words in your head about using do not move your hands—unless you want them to move.

For example, tell yourself to stand up. Have no intention of standing up, just say the words in your mind. Did thinking the words make you stand up when you did not want to? Words in your head do not directly control your actions. They are just symbols that pass through your mind if you do not buy into them. They will be there. Why fight them to go away when you can just accept them as being there and control your hands instead of the words in your head.

Ready for another exercise? Try to discover cues in your environment that make you feel like drinking or using drugs. When you discover something that makes you feel like drinking or drugging, how long can you keep your value decision while in the presence of the cue? For example, I keep a glass pipe used to smoke crack cocaine and amphetamines and a mirror with a razor blade in a paper bag for some to use as a cue. Someone focuses on his or her plan to never again use. I bring out the bag and shake it. For many, as soon as they hear the glass mirror and pipe jingling in the bag, they report that they feel like using. I put away the bag. Make room for the feeling to use. Understand it can return at any time. Do not fight its presence. Return to your value decision and focus on it. Continue the exercise until you can look at the drug paraphernalia and feel the value decision while controlling your hands.

Rather than run, accept the feelings and ideas to use. People who want to quit marijuana can use plastic bags, pipes, and rolling papers. People who inject can be presented with syringes, needles, or junky works. Drinkers can look at glasses and bottles of alcohol. The end result is to have the decision live with cues to drink alcohol or use drugs. You don't have to discover all your cues, because cues do not trigger your hands to move. Cues may stimulate your primitive brain to make you think about and feel like drinking or drugging, but they do not trigger your hands to move. You control your hands. If viewing the cues leaves you with an aftereffect, use your decision to quit forever to know what you are going to do. Accept your thoughts and feelings to use as being present, because they are. Make room for the thoughts and feelings about drinking alcohol and use drugs to be present at some time. Whenever they are present, that is when they should cross your mind. Nothing to worry about because they are just thoughts and sensations you let pass without buying into them with meaning. That is what we talk about at Quitting Forever meetings.

Are you ready for another exercise? Imagine your life now that you no longer drink alcohol or use drugs. Where will you go, and what will you do? Ordinary life experiences are rituals and celebrations. Imagine the office party after work with an open bar. Will you always want to avoid going to the party just because alcohol will be served? What about a New Year's party or your birthday?

Remember as many things as you can that you liked to do while drinking alcohol or using drugs. Now, imagine yourself doing those activities without drinking or drugging. Include in your imagery the scene of feeling like or having the experience of remembering the fun of using and drinking and use your decision about never using to gain the upper hand. Imagine doing those activities without drinking or drugging, and learn to enjoy them just because they are fun.

Are you ready for another exercise? This is a twist to the former exercise. Life is filled with unpleasant things. We lose friends and loved ones. People die. We try to do something, and we fail at the task. People get reprimanded at jobs. People get rejected in dating and mating. Sometimes we feel tired or even depressed. We get lonely. Things anger us. Imagine some unpleasant things happening to you. List a few events that have happened and a few likely to happen. What are you most afraid of happening? Imagine any of these things, and see yourself abstaining from alcohol or drugs. Let yourself acknowledge how it would be possible to feel like or think about using alcohol or drugs at those times. Use your skill of saying to yourself, "*never.*" See yourself controlling your hands. See yourself as someone who never uses alcohol or drugs. That is who you are now. What you are doing is more than a set of words you say to yourself.

Are you ready for another exercise? How might someone talk you into using alcohol or drugs? Where would you be? Invent a scene as real to life that you can imagine. First, how would you use your decision about never using? Second, how would you use your decision to talk to the person trying to get you to use? Talk about as many refusal strategies as you can imagine even if they are serious, rude, silly or absurd.

Imagination is fine for practice, but you are going to have to live your life as someone who never uses alcohol or drugs. Go out and do anything you want, and go wherever you want. People who don't use alcohol or drugs do not have to avoid places because they do not use. They can go wherever they want, because they can keep themselves from using alcohol or drugs. If you find yourself feeling like avoiding someplace because you might drink or use, you are maintaining abstinence and perhaps have not quit forever. What is it about that place that makes you think you might use there? You talk about that at a Quitting Forever meeting. You have not finished quitting forever until you are 100 percent sure you will never drink or use drugs—no matter what happens or no matter where you go. It is time to use your skill and use it strongly. Face your doubts.

Want to make sure you will keep your decision to abstain from alcohol or drugs forever? Revisit your decision to never drink or use alcohol. When you made the decision, did you make it final? A way of finalizing your decision is to recognize you might think of changing that decision. Now, say to yourself, "The subject of changing the decision is over. The decision is not open for discussion or negotiation. I will never change my mind on this decision. Not only will I never drink or drug again, but I will never change the decision to never drink or drug again because it is more than words in my head and abstaining is something I do. I want a final resolution to my quitting forever, and the only way that will happen is if I never drink or drug again. The only way I will never drink or drug again is if I make it happen. I decided it would happen. I decide I will never re-decide by deliberating. The subject of whether or not I will drink or use drugs is closed in my mind. The debate is over."

## Deliberating and Changing Your Mind

A decision to quit forever is all you need to abstain for the remainder of your life—unless you go back on your values. Some people are cavalier about their decision to abstain forever. With a cavalier attitude, it is easy to dismiss important matters. If you find it easy to dismiss your decision, you feel little remorse when you return to your former drinking or drugging. If you drink or drug again, and it doesn't bother you at all that you went against your decision and broke your word to yourself, you probably will have some difficulty using decision-based abstinence.

Quitting forever using decision-based abstinence is for people who want to be self-responsible. Part of self-responsibility is admitting to yourself when you fall short of your goal and feel dissatisfied. You don't have to hate yourself for what you have done; I have talked with too many people who hated themselves because they drank or used again. Many of those people used the feeling of self-hate to convince themselves drinking and using was not the thing to do again and went on to permanent exit and quitting forever. Other people just hated that they drank or used drugs again. They only hated what they had done, not themselves, and continued their decision, returning to abstinence and never drank or used drugs again.

Other people quit forever and use the skill but fall back to reasoning. They begin by saying that they will never again use, and then follow that with reasons to abstain. The reasons to abstain are usually countered in their mind with reasons to drink and drug, and deliberation has started. For example, your old drinking friend returns to town and comes over to your house with his best home-brewed beer. Your friend tells you he is moving to the other side of the country and will not likely be brewing beer again. He wants you to take part in this last chance to drink his last batch of home brew with him. Your friend reminds you of all the good times you had together, and there is only one quart of beer for the both of you. One quart for two people is not enough to intoxicate you. Nothing bad will happen if you drink with your friend. You use your skill and say to yourself, "I never drink anymore." But, you really feel like having a drink under these circumstances. You hear yourself thinking, *But this will not hurt you. This is your last chance. Do you really want to offend a friend who is going away?* Instead of letting these words just be there, you buy into them and say to yourself, "It will hurt me if I start drinking again." You hear in your mind, "No, it will not. How can you be sure? Just a little bit one more time will not make a difference."

Recognize how two sides of a debate are set. As soon as you went beyond never, you were in a point-counterpoint argument and debate with yourself. Examine the debate. It seems like ambivalence. "Should I drink, or should I abstain?" That is the debate. Why would you debate whether or not you should drink again if you have quit forever. Deciding to quit forever means ending the debate. Nevertheless, people who decided on quitting forever have told me they found themselves engaged in an internal debate. Some people experience the debate like bargaining. Debating or bargaining are both like ambivalence; your mind is not made up. You are deliberating whether you should drink or use drugs.

What can you do when you discover you are debating yourself about whether to drink alcohol and/or use drugs? Recognize you are debating or bargaining and say, "I am choosing whether or not I will drink or use drugs." Then, ask yourself, "If I am done quitting forever, why am I debating?" But, if you finished quitting forever, you know your mind is made up. Let the debate be a bunch of words you observe. They are just words going back and forth: point and counterpoint. Step away from the debate and observe it while not being part of it. Let the drinking debate go on. There is no winning or losing with just a bunch of words. Return to your decision, "I never drink alcohol or use drugs." You do not have to control your mind when you control your hands.

How do you feel now that you decided not to drink or use drugs and had an abstinence experience? Was your self-confidence shaken because you caught yourself debating? If you caught yourself, you know you can recognize a return to debating about drinking or drugging. There is a risk only if you are maintaining abstinence and have not made a permanent exit from alcohol and/or drug use.

Some people continue to choose whether they will drink. They continue to figure out whether they will drink or use drugs. They count time and make a big deal about how long they have not drank or used drugs. These people have not made a permanent exit, no matter how long they have not drank or used drugs. If they don't feel like drinking or drugging, then they do not do it. But, as soon as they feel like it or when there are alcohol and/or drugs around, they return to choosing and the debating and bargaining starts again. They may get good at their debating, but they have not made a permanent exit. A chance remains they will lose the debate and bargain for drinking and/or drugging and then choose to drink or use.

Once you use and sober up or come down from the high, you again are faced with thinking about quitting forever. If you are not thinking about quitting forever, then you are open to drinking alcohol or using drugs. We have already gone over some of the many problems caused by alcohol and drugs. It will very likely be just a matter of time before you have the problems drinking or drug use cause. At that time—or before—you may think about whether you should quit forever. It is never too late. Keep quitting forever until you carry it out. Quitting forever is something everyone can do once they make up their mind. How made up is your mind? What risks do you want to take with your life? You never again have to risk having the problems caused by drinking or using. You can quit forever.

# How to Keep Yourself from Drinking or Drugging

Don't do anything to keep yourself from drinking or drugging other than to abstain. But, now that you will never drink alcohol or use drugs again, what are you going to do with the time you have? Do whatever else it is you want to do. Don't say to yourself, "I am going to the gym so

I won't drink or use drugs." That is not facing your responsibility about quitting forever. Say to yourself, "Since I no longer drink or use drugs, I have extra time to go to the gym now. So, even though I may feel like using alcohol or drugs, I will never use them because of quitting forever. Since I won't be using alcohol or drugs, I will use this time to go to the gym." It is a very real difference. You are keeping yourself from drinking by following your values more than distracting yourself by doing something so you will not think about or have time for drinking or drugging. You are following your values, not what passes through your mind.

Distraction works in the short run. So, you say to yourself, "I feel like drinking, and I will avoid it by doing something else and distracting myself from the feeling to drink. Then, I won't have to think about drinking or using drugs." It works, but for how long? Plus, it does another thing. If you only use distraction, it keeps you from facing your real responsibility. When it comes to future drinking or drugging, your responsibility to yourself is to follow your values. If you don't know what you are going to do, you haven't found your values. What is important to you?

What happens is people use distraction and count time. Then, they say to themselves, "I haven't drank or drugged in six months," or whatever amount of time, and they conclude, "I don't want to break that streak." But, it does not get them to face the issue of whether they will do it again. Some people carry out that streak of not doing it for a long time, and some say that it has been so long since they used that they would never do it again. You can do it that way, but the risk of using over time is increased because you didn't say you would never do it again; that came later. You can say to yourself, "Now I will never drink again," whenever you decide. But, sooner or later, it becomes test time. Test time is when there is a drinking opportunity, and you have to figure out what you are going to do. You either will drink and drug or not drink and drug. Are you going to take the test?

Other people think of the bad consequences of drinking or drug use to talk themselves out of doing it. That is the relapse-prevention approach. But, bringing up bad things that will happen is like a bargain or an argument. Reasons not to drink or use are one side of the argument. But, if you can be convinced the bad things will not happen, that is the other side of the argument and quite a bargain. Why not drink or use if you can get away with it? Maybe you can get away with it this time. You never said you would never drink again. You just don't want those things that happened in the past to happen again. Well, maybe this time they won't happen. This time it will be different. You don't have a car to drive. You are in another town, and the next two days are a holiday with a vacation. Other people are partying and getting loaded. No one will even notice you are loaded too, and you have plenty of time to sober up and come down afterward. That is the counterargument to always having to remember consequences. It is bargaining if you can get away without bad consequences. You always know that it is only a risk that bad consequences may happen, but it also means that they may not happen. Do you want to keep bargaining your way out of your next drink or drug use?

## Explicit Instruction: Making Your Decision

I offer you a way to make your decision if you have not yet made it. It is time for a decisive engagement about what you are doing. Say to yourself right now, "What will it be, will I ever drink or use drugs again?" If you don't answer that question, then you can't finish quitting forever. If you say, "I won't do it for right now," you leave the door open for later use, possibly the next time. Some people say, "I don't have a plan to drink or drug again." And, that may be true. But, having no plan to drink or drug and having a made a decision not to drink or drug are two different things. No plan to drink just means drinking or drug use is not on your mind right now. A decision not to drink means that, if it is on your mind you won't do it. Waiting until it is on your mind is the hardest time to figure out what to do. You are biased at that time. Maybe it is even a physical influence because you feel like doing it. You will be face to face with your conditioning due to alcohol and drug use. That is why you are better off having your mind made up ahead of time. That is why your decision about quitting forever works so well.

You would do better not to make yourself think about consequences. Distracting yourself can be a way to avoid your internal experience when it would be better to observe. Instead of thinking about consequences or distracting yourself from the thoughts and feeling to use, make quitting forever an event that happened. As an event, it becomes a reference point to anchor your value. It was a day of decision. You stopped trying to control your thoughts and feelings to use, and you stopped running from them. You accepted them for what they were as the result of using and started controlling your hands.

Now, when you feel like it, you know you completed quitting forever, because it is something you have already done. Since you have already finished quitting forever, there is nothing to consider. There is nothing more to figure out. There is nothing to do but control your hands. The thoughts and feelings about drinking alcohol or using drugs do not have to be countered with consequences. You do not have to use distraction to hide from your reaction. Develop a willingness to observe your reactions, making peace with them as you watch words and sensations, harmless mind chatter and body changes that you know your mind and body sometimes does after quitting forever. Accept what is going on inside you as part of the natural process of quitting forever. There is nothing to be worried about. You control your hands.

The reasons for quitting forever and the reason why you are not drinking are two different things. The reason you are not drinking is because you decided not do it anymore, and you would never change your mind. The promise you made is a decision for action not a set of words you have to remember. You made your mind up that way. A decision never to drink alcohol or use drugs is an internal thing that is a little bit different for everyone. The person quitting forever may not always completely understand how the decision was made. But, you know quitting forever is done because you know that your drinking and drugging is over. Once the jump is made, you can't un-jump. You will always control your hands and abstain from drink and drugs not buying into thoughts questioning your decision or being concerned that you still have thoughts or feelings about drinking and drugging again sometimes. You may not know many of the reasons why you quit forever, but you it was done.

The reason you will never drink again is because of quitting forever. Once you are abstaining because you decided you would, you made up your mind. A predetermined decision is the way you are going to do it. At that point, it is impossible to talk yourself out of abstaining if you stopped bargaining or arguing or running and hiding. If you use quitting forever as your sole reason, you now don't drink or use drugs because you made the decision not to do it anymore. The reasons why you made the decision are unimportant.

Quitting forever is what you did for yourself. Your own hard work and your own good thinking—and very little else—got you here. When it comes to quitting forever, no one but you can make it happen. Other people can talk to you about it, but no one can make you carry it out. You can be kept from alcohol and drugs by going into inpatient treatment or having the legal system watch over you. That is temporary. You have to figure out on your own if quitting forever is for you to carry out, and a certain amount of that process is just intuitive. You can know quitting forever was carried out when you control your hands, know you always will abstain, and feel good about not drinking and using drugs.

Get out there and get going with your life. Now that you are not drinking and drugging, work on the things important to you. You don't have to do anything special. Once you're not drinking or drugging, you can live your life the way you want, and without alcohol or drugs.

## Someone After Quitting Forever Drank and Used Again

I know someone who wanted to quit forever and went to Quitting Forever, and they drank or used drugs again. So, how can you say you will never drink or use drugs again?

Going to meetings or therapy sessions does nothing to a person that they do not do to themselves. The fact the person drank or used drugs means nothing more than individual choice was exercised although the choice may have some harmful results. What about all the people who attended sessions and never drank again? The fact that people went to a meeting to learn about quitting forever and never drank again also means nothing, since going to a meeting does nothing than help with misunderstanding when someone is seeking clarification on what they read. A person does something to himself or herself. We are talking about a person's ability to decide abstinence and carry out the decision.

The issue is not whether a person went to what meeting, but whether a person will quit forever—and if the individual has quit forever. The fact that people from all walks of life, and with all levels of alcohol and drug problems, quit forever is well established. Remember, in its publication *Grapevine*, AA admitted that 60 percent of the people who have stopped drinking do so outside of Twelve-Step attendances.

Why would one person drinking or not drinking [drugging or not drugging] become a prediction of how another person is going to do? If a person goes to twelve-step groups and works a good program but yet drinks, is twelve-step attendance questioned? No, the person is sent back for more twelve-step recovery. If a person claims to never want to drink again yet goes against his or her best interest and drinks, does that mean the individual should give up the idea of permanent exit by decision-based abstinence from drunkenness or being high? No, the person should be able to learn what he or she did to self-defeat and then return to decision-based abstinence. So, with decision-based abstinence, the question is not really about attending anything. Decision-based abstinence is something an individual carries out. The question to be addressed is whether the person has the intent for permanent, decision-based abstinence.

Why would anyone discourage a person who drank alcohol or used drugs from carrying out permanent abstinence? What would be the purpose? Engage in an analogy. I am not doing something I want to do that will benefit me and make a positive change in my life. Therefore, I go to a counselor to help me. The counselor spends time convincing me that I cannot do the thing I want to do. Why bother to go to counseling? I already know I have not been making the beneficial change. Not making the change is discouraging enough. I am looking for assistance to overcome that limitation. I am asking for help to be able to do something positive. I am now being told that because I did not do it, I cannot do it. And because I cannot do it, I should give up. Why are you discouraging me from wanting to make a positive change in my life by never doing something again? Saying it cannot be done goes against the evidence of that people have done it. Where is the evidence that I am not one of those people? Anyone can say I cannot, but where is the evidence?

The confusion is from misunderstanding statistics. Suppose 25 percent of the people studied drank again after quitting forever. Would that mean that you have a 25 percent chance of drinking again after quitting forever? No. There is a difference between you and a group. Quitting forever is something any person can carry out. If the person next to you changes their mind and drinks, how does that increase your chances of drinking? If the person drank again, that means he or she did not quit forever, because quitting forever means you do not change your mind. Does that mean you are going to change your mind? That would be like saying your mind is controlled by someone other than you. Some substance abuse counselors have said to me, "if you see someone drink who said they quit forever drinking or using drugs than, it would have an influence on you." If seeing someone else quit forever and then drinking or drugging influences you, then you have not quit forever, because quitting forever means not changing your mind about never drinking or using drugs even if someone else changes his or her mind.

Understand the difference between dependant events and independent events. A deck of cards is the best example. If there are fifty-two cards in the deck, the chance of drawing an ace of spades is one in fifty-two. With dependent events, the chance of drawing an ace of spades after the first card is drawn is one in fifty-one. With independent events, the first card drawn is reentered into the deck, so with each draw the odds of drawing an ace of spades remain one in fifty-two.

Bring it back to you being affected by someone else's drinking or drugging after quitting forever. You are never going to drink or use drugs again. You know how to recognize a change of mind and use your ability to control your hands to keep from drinking and drugging. You have kept yourself from drinking/drugging before and are 100 percent confident that you will never drink or drug again. Someone else's drinking is an independent event from you. Because you expected others to drink and use drugs, the chance of your confidence being shaken is zero. You knew that other people would return to drinking after saying they quit forever. Just because they let themselves down does not mean that you are going to let yourself down. You know your decision to abstain is based on you alone. The chances of you drinking or drugging again are the same before seeing someone else drink or drug than after you witness it. And, if someone who wants to quit forever drinks again, that person's chances of quitting forever are the same after they drank as they were before. If someone intends to quit forever, they will succeed if they keep quitting until it is forever. Quitting and maintaining abstinence and permanent exit by quitting forever are two different events.

The fact is people are quitting forever, and for good, all the time. When they quit using alcohol and drugs, they look like ordinary people with ordinary problems they struggle to solve in a sober state of mind. If you have quit forever, it is not for you to prove that you will never drink again. Your behavior is proof. The ones who say you will drink are discouraging you. Where is the evidence that you will drink again if you are not drinking or using drugs now, and if you claim you will carry out that decision for the remainder of your life? If having once done something meant a person was doomed to do it again forever, why would there be any need for counseling, groups, or meetings to bring about change?

Get it the first time around—or after that. People who don't succeed in quitting forever the first time eventually do succeed in quitting forever if they continue the natural process. Or they give up and keep drinking and drugging themselves to death. Some people return to the recovery movement and the twelve steps, where they can get support for their relapsing. Where do you want to be next year. You can be sitting in a recovery group calling yourself an alcoholic or an addict, or you can end all that by quitting forever. It is up to what you do with your hands.

# Life Goes On

Life goes on with you not drinking or using drugs after quitting forever. You do not need to do anything to recover from alcohol and drug abuse other than to never drink alcohol and se drugs for the remainder of your life. Once you quit forever, you are indistinguishable from everyone else in America. You have the same life tasks and problems—both practical and emotional—as everyone else in your situation. Examples of life tasks are where you are going to live, how you are going to support yourself, what your family and social life look like, what you want to learn, how you are going to care for your health, and legal matters.

Practical problems arise when you try to accomplish life tasks and you cannot get what you want. Emotional problems arise when you have an emotional reaction to not getting what you want in life. Facing life tasks and having practical and emotional problems will not make you drink or use drugs after quitting forever. You face problems to try to get more of what you want and less of what you don't want. You have your own natural limitations, which are based on your biology, learning ability, and available resources. There is still plenty you can do, but you do not have to do anything to recover other than abstain forever.

You may have legal or personal reasons to continue Quitting Forever after quitting forever. People who have quit forever sometimes realize how easy it is to accomplish. Do you want to take part in telling others about the natural process of quitting forever? You can be part of meeting where you talk with people about quitting forever. Do you have legal issues where someone is forcing you to attend twelve-step groups against your will? Contact me at the www.quittingforever.org, or call (775) 786-8801. I will assist you in setting up some Quitting Forever discussion meetings that will count for your court-mandated twelve-step groups.

Even though you never drink or use drugs again, you may have some aftereffects because of what you have done to yourself. Do you have issues left over as the result of your drinking or drugging? A major issue people have talked about is others not believing they have quit forever.

People who do not believe you will express their disbelief with either positive or negative emotions. Friends who want you to drink or drug with them may laugh at you when you tell them you don't drink or drug. They may take a condescending stance and guffaw as they say, "Sure you aren't going to drink or drug anymore." You may be at a loss as to what to say in this situation, even though you are not going to drink or use drugs.

Family members may distrust you. When family members feel anxiety because you are late or due to interpersonal conflict, they may accuse you of drinking or drugging again. Your family may be living with resentment about the way you acted when you were drinking and drugging and hold it against you. You may witness yelling, crying, and displays of anger by your family members that results from the way you treated them when you were loaded. You will likely feel some strong emotions yourself when confronted with strong emotional displays.

You don't necessarily have to have aftereffects from your drinking and drugging, but if you do, admit it to yourself and accept them as something caused by your drinking and drug use. If you never use again, the aftereffects will resolve themselves over time. The time it takes for resolution varies, and you might be able to move resolution along. How you do that is up to you. One way is to use your creative skills at interpersonal problem solving. You might try to work things out with people on a one-to-one basis. Calling a family meeting can work toward resolution. Be patient with the people who are upset with you about the way you acted in the past. Accept that they have a reason to be upset with you. Assure them that you will not be drinking or drugging anymore, but you will have to prove it to them by carrying out what you assured them by never drinking or drugging—no matter what happens. You can make that promise because you have the skill and you know how to use it. Some marriage and family therapists are natural about twelve-step attendance. They may be able to help you resolve family and interpersonal matters.

Beware if you seek help from any therapist as some use a twelve step counseling model without telling you before you sit down with them in a session. The twelve-step movement has influenced many therapists. If you seek out a therapist, ask them if they use the twelve steps. Alanon is twelve steps for families. Alanon maintains that alcoholism and drug addiction is a family disease. They also are confused about cause and effect. The Alanon concept is that your family is equally responsible as you are for your drinking and drugging. Instead, your family has been impacted by your alcohol and/or drug use. The degree and extent of that impact varies from family to family. The impact of your drinking and drugging on the family did not cause you to drink or use drugs. You alone are responsible for what you have done.

If the counselor or therapist denies being twelve-step-oriented, you might try them, but beware. If they lied and start talking twelve steps in a session, excuse yourself and your family and announce you will leave. Contact me, and I will assist you in filing a complaint with the counselor's licensing agency. I will contact the counselor by letter and phone to voice a complaint. We may consider legal action if you care to pursue it.

Single people wonder how they will mingle and find a partner now that they are not drinking or drugging. Meeting someone for romantic and sexual relations is one of life's tasks. Alcohol or drugs lower anxiety in social situations, while acquiring and consuming alcohol and/or drugs become a shared activity.

If you are single and interested in meeting someone for romantic interests, you have a better chance of finding the type of relationship you were looking for now that you never drink or use drugs. You can take the time you used thinking about and using alcohol and/or drugs and use it to find someone you can approach. You will learn a lot about yourself and other people by trying to find someone just for you. The best way to meet people is through friends, so keep meeting new people and making friends. Let people know you are single and looking to meet someone for more than a friendship. Wherever people meet is a good place to meet someone.

If you are married or in a serious relationship, you have an opportunity to rekindle the kind of relationship you would like to have. Relationships work best when you work at them. Now that you are not preoccupied with alcohol and/or drugs, you can reexamine your relationship with your husband, wife, or significant other. If you have children, you can spend more time with them. Remember, alcohol and/or drugs have been your other love. Your love is divided when you are drinking and using. You don't need a recovery support group. You would be better off getting love and support from your family and friends. In support groups, they give you support so you will not drink alcohol and/or use drugs. Without support groups, you don't drink alcohol and/or use drugs. so you can engage your family. The way to get support is to give support. Reengage your family.

Reengaging family is not for everyone. Resolving an alcohol and drug problem confident about never using again leaves some aware of the fact that they do not want to be in the relationship. I have known people who finally left an abusive family situation because they were no longer drunk or high. You can decide to end a useless relationship. If you are stuck, a marriage and family or couples therapist may be of help to you.

What about family members who continue to drink or use drugs? Your choice is to tolerate them, fight with them about what they are doing, reason with them, or leave the situation. You are under no obligation to help anyone else quit alcohol and/or drugs forever. Everyone is responsible for his or her own behavior. Do not get involved in the intervention movement, or you will be backing twelve-step treatment. You might issue an ultimatum: tell that family member he or she better do something about getting drunk or getting high. Stop making excuses for others. When the family member is drunk or high, openly tell them and anyone who asks about him or her. For instance, rather than give them an excuse, tell a caller that the family member is too drunk or high to come to the phone. A competent marriage and family/couples therapist, mental health counselor, or psychologist who is neutral about twelve-step attendance may be helpful, but remember my caution.

Your professional carriers or jobs will likely benefit when you quit forever. Your job attendance will probably improve. On Mondays and after holidays, you will not be hung over or coming down from a runner. That will give you advantages over employees who still drink and use. Contact me if your employer insists you should attend AA or NA meetings as a contingency of employment.

Religious people who have stopped practicing their religion have a chance to repent. Free will and forgiveness are the cornerstones of Christian religious faith. You can use your free will to keep yourself from doing the wrong thing. If you decided it is wrong for you to be get drunk or high on drugs, it can be of benefit to your spiritual life. Repentance is where you say you are sorry for doing the wrong thing and ask forgiveness because you will no longer do the wrong thing. Is it time to reengage with your church group, or do you want to explore other church groups? The Jewish or Islamic community will welcome you if you seek them. This is America, and although not everyone honors freedom of religion, you are still free to seek out the religious community of your choice, or not attend at all.

The Jewish Torah advises purification through abstention from alcohol. Other religious faiths do not condone drinking. Islam excludes alcohol. Alcohol is what is called Haram in Islam. Buddhists teach that alcohol and drugs interfere with the quest to understand and develop the mind. Hinduism has the expectation that devotees will avoid alcohol and drugs. If you are going to follow the religion of your choice, you can get plenty of support and be part of a community.

There is American Atheist and Secular Humanism if you are atheist or humanist. Many communities have secular groups getting together. You can find them by using the Internet. Your purpose in attending is to meet like-minded people, not to keep yourself from drinking or drugging. You keep yourself from drinking and/or drugging because of quitting forever.

You don't change your life to keep from using alcohol and drugs. Your life changes after quitting forever the use of alcohol and drugs as the result of quitting forever. Problems haven't caused you to drink alcohol or use drugs. Alcohol and drugs caused problems. What made you drink or use drugs was that you had used them in the past. Then, you ran to the high when you had problems, to celebrate, and when you were bored. You drank alcohol and used drugs when bad things happened, when good things happened, and when nothing happened. You were not running away from a problem; you were running to get high. All of that is over now. Now, you will face problems or ignore them, celebrate or humbug, and sit around bored or find something to amuse yourself all without drinking or using drugs.

What will you do with your life after quitting forever, when alcohol and drugs are no longer part of your life? Imagine how you want it to be next year, five years, and ten years from now. Where do you want to be living? With what friends and family do you want to be associating? What do you want to learn? What kind of work would you like to be doing? Your life will change as the result of not drinking alcohol and/or using drugs. You can just let things happen, or you can take charge of your life and try to make some things happen. When you try something new, you can never be sure of the outcome. That can be exciting or make you feel insecure.

When you feel insecure about the future and how difficult it is to accomplish many of life's tasks, you know you can be secure about one thing as life becomes stressful and unpredictable, you know one thing you can always count on. After quitting forever, you know you will never drink alcohol and use drugs for the remainder of your life. During insecure times, when you have little control over other people and your life situation, you can always draw comfort in knowing no matter what happens, you will never get drunk or stoned on drugs.

# Court Ruling Finding AA/NA Twelve-Step to be Religious Activity

June 5, 2007; United Stated Court of Appeals for the Ninth Circuit. No. 06-15474; D.C. No. CV-04-00026-DAE Opinion: Ricky K. Inouye Plaintiff.

April 10, 2001; United States District Court, Eastern District of Wisconsin: Bausch, Plaintiff versus Sumiec, Sullivan and Litchcher.

March 29, 2001; United States District Court for Northern District of Illinois Eastern Division; Manning versus United Airlines.

February 4, 1998; Equal Employment Opportunity Commission; Manning versus United Airlines.

May 14, 1997; United State Courts of Appeals; Warner versus Orange County Department of Probation.

November 10, 1997; Supreme Court of Tennessee; Evans versus Board of Paroles.

June 11, 1996; New York Court of Appeals; Evans versus Board of Paroles.

August, 1996; U.S. Court of Appeals, Seventh District; Kerr versus Lind, et al.

For review of court cases finding AA/NA Twelve Steps religious:

Columbia Law Review: 97 Colum. L. Rev. 437 (1997) Michael G. Honeymar, Jr. Alcoholics Anonymous as a Condition of Drunk Driving Probation: When Does It Amount to Establishment of Religion.

Duke Law Journal (Feb 1998) Volume 47 Number 4, p.785: Derek P. Apanovitch. Religion and Rehabilitation: The Requisition of God by the State.

**How to resist if the court is attempting to sentence you to AA or NA**

1 Agree to attend AA and NA as the judge sentenced.

2. Ask for the court to record that your First Amendment right of freedom of religion is being violated.

3. Provide the court with a list of the above rulings, and ask that it be placed in the court record they received a list of court rulings finding AA/NA religious.

4. Get a copy of the court records.

5. Contact a lawyer and file a lawsuit. Contact Quitting Forever (775) 786-8801; www.quittingforever.org.

# References

Bufe, Charles (1991) *Alcoholics Anonymous: Cult or Cure?* See Sharp Press: San Francisco.

Ellis, Albert, and Velten, Emmett (1992) *When AA Doesn't Work for You: Rational Steps to Quitting Alcohol.* Barricade Books: Fort Lee, New Jersey.

Fransway, Rebecca (2000) *12 Step Horror Stories: True Tales of Misery, Betrayal, and Abuse in AA, NA, and 12 Step Treatment.* See Sharp Press: Tucson, Arizona.

Hayes, Steven C., Strosahl, Kirk D., and Wilson, Kelly G. (2003) *Acceptance and Commitment Therapy: An Experiential Approach to Behavior Change.* Guilford Press: New York.

Miller, William R. (1999) *Enhancing Motivation for Change in Substance Abuse Treatment.* U.S. Department of Health and Human Services, Public Health Service, Substance Abuse and Mental Health Services Administration Center for Substance Abuse Treatment: Rockville, Maryland.

Maultsby, Maxie C. (1978) *The Rational Behavioral Alcohol-Relapse Prevention Treatment Method.* Rational Self-Help Aid, Inc: Lexington, Kentucky.

Peele, Stanton, and Bufe, Charles, with Brodsky, Archie (2000) *Resisting 12 Step Coercion: How to Fight Forced Participation in AA, NA, or 12 Step Treatment.* See Sharp Press: Tucson, Arizona.

Peele, Stanton (1989) Diseasing of America: Addiction Treatment Out of Control. Lexington Books, D.C. Hearth and Company, Lexington, Massachusetts.

Trimpey, Jack (1994) *The Final Fix for Alcohol and Drug Addiction: AVRT: Addictive Voice Recognition Technique.* Lotus Press: Lotus, California.

# Notes